A Woman's Tell,
A True Story

"Worries"

Sitting, in my room confused and in pain,
Softly, wishing relief from my burdens,
Hiding beneath the covers of guilt,
Wondering will the truths come out,
Will the doors once closed become open,
Hoping, that I can travel those roads left untraveled,
Finally, breaking the circles that have continued throughout my life.

To order additional copies of this book, contact:
Xlibris Corporation
1-888-795-4274
www.Xlibris.com
Orders@Xlibris.com
99768

Chapter One

I can relate to many teenage moms, because I am one. Girls pay close attention to this story; it just may save you from being a teenage mom, and learn a few life lessons along the way. If you are one then I hope you can find the faith, hope, and strength I have. Never give up and work to be the best mom you can be. My name is Evelyn and here is my story. It started the summer of 1987 when I was 7; I had all these feeling in me about this boy named Ethan. I wanted to be with him. I thought he was cute. Ethan, his brother, and I had been swimming all day. They were hungry when we made it to my aunt Dorothy's house. I knew how to cook fries and they didn't. I told him that I would cook them some if he liked me. He said he did so I cooked for them. When they finished eating Ethan and I started making out. My aunt's boyfriend caught us and told my aunt on us. My mom told me I need to stop being sexual and be a kid, because it could lead to me getting pregnant. She had enough kids to know that I wouldn't want to deal with the pain of child birth and I wasn't ready to handle the responsibilities that come along with being a mom. We didn't stop, we just became more careful. He ended up moving and we didn't see each other on a regular basis. It was 1990 when Ethan and his brother Garrett started to come to our house again on the weekends. I felt I was in love with him, but I was afraid to tell him. I ended up telling his brother how I felt. He told him and come to find out he liked me too. Ethan came to me one day and said his brother told him what I said. We talked about dating each other. We decided we had to keep our relationship secret, because his mom was dating my uncle Larry. At first we just talked until one day he wanted to feel my body. I didn't tell him no, because I wanted him too. I didn't tell him at that time he broke my virginity. He couldn't tell, because there wasn't that much blood. The next week I was scared I was pregnant, because when he pulled out he was shooting sperm and we didn't use protection. I began to relax when I talked to my friends and they told me if I hadn't started my period I didn't have anything to worry about.(I didn't have long to relax about having unprotected sex, because I started my period a few days after my 11th birthday.

A few months after I lost my virginity.) He made me feel so special so it wasn't hard to forget about the pregnancy scare. After awhile it became something we did on a regular basis. We weren't so smart to use protection all the time. Since, we had a secret relationship I felt couldn't get mad when he was out dating other girls. I thought no one would pay attention to our relationship if I let him keep flirting with girls like he always has. I was an honor roll student I had to keep my grades up and made sure I never missed school, so no one would suspect I had other things going on. It was now 1992 and the only one that noticed something was going on was my dad. My mom worked 2 jobs to take care of us, so she was at work or too tired to notice. My dad noticed what was going on, because we always argued and stayed mad at each other. It was ok for him to go places and hang out with girls, but he didn't want me going places or talking to boys. So we argued about it. As time went on I felt our feeling for each other grew. In a way I was right, but in another he just wanted me for the sex. I didn't realize this right off, because we would sit and spilled our hearts out to one another. I felt sorry for him, because he had so many dreams and hopes, and he had no one to help him achieve them. He would cry to me when we were alone. His mom couldn't afford to buy him, his brother or sister things, because she was busy with her life. She did not pay attention to theirs. I don't know if she didn't want to work or couldn't work to provide for them better than she did. I also didn't know until later why she was so intent on making her relationship with my uncle Larry work. Maybe I was the only person he could talk to who wouldn't judge or make fun of him, because of the way he lived at the time. While Ethan and Garrett were spending the weekend at my house their mom went to jail, I can't remember what for, but my uncle Larry was in jail too. Ethan and his brother was staying with us until his mom made arrangements for them to live with someone else until she or my uncle got out. One afternoon my brother Derek, my sisters Karen and Mary, my cousin Jamie and I went with them to their house. My dad wanted us to see if there was someone who could take care of them at their house. When we got there, there was this boy who was the neighborhood bully standing at the end of their street with a long pole. He wanted to hurt Ethan and Garrett. He and his friends were always waiting to catch them at home alone. This particular day the bully wanted to hurt them more than he ever had. He chased us with this big, long pole. He became enraged, because we were too fast for him to catch us. When we made it in the house everybody was laughing and talking about the incident that no one, but me kept watching the bully through the screen door. Ethan was standing in front of the door inside the house. Before I knew it the bully threw the pole through the screen of the door. I saw the pole coming and I dived on Ethan. He thought I was angry and pushed him. I told him I wasn't mad I saw the boy throwing the pole. I then pointed to the pole. It was sticking in the wall where his head had been. Later on when, we made it *back to my house, he told me how much he loved me and was thankful I saved his life. We grew a little closer. One of our favorite games to play was to see who would fall asleep first. After the person fell asleep We would do what we wanted to them while they were asleep. My brother, sisters, my cousin Jamie, Ethan, Garrett, and I would walk to the grocery store at 1 or 2 in the morning. To have a party. If we weren't doing those things we would swim until one in the morning. The neighbors always had something to complain to my mom about, because we would play jokes on them or each other. When Ethan and I were around other kids, we had codes. One of us would point the bad finger or say f*** you and the other would whisper when. We would say it when no one was paying attention. Then make plans to meet. When we could Ethan and I would sneak away. There were these apartments next to ours. The hallways upstairs had these walls, which made the area by the window look like a small room. We would hide there and have sex so we could hear when my brother, sisters, and his brother were looking for us. Since I had started my period I was afraid to have sex with him without protection. I didn't want him to be angry at me and the best part for me was we were with each other, so I didn't say anything. He in a roundabout way went back to his old self when summer ended and his mom came home.*

Chapter Two

The fall of 1992 had come. That school year I rarely saw Ethan at first. He was dating other girls and I was still being the model student. There were boys interested in me, but I loved him too much to date them. I only saw him when he and my brother got together to meet girls on certain weekends. Him messing with other girls started taking its toll on me and I began to tell him I wasn't dating other boys, so why was he dating other girls? He would always convince me that he had to so no one would notice us. He was quite the smooth talker. Out of the blue his mom asked me to spend the weekend at her house, because she was tired of being the only female in the house. Ethan's sister had gotten married and moved out. I went over to their house, because she and I were close. When Ethan found out I was coming he decided to stay home. When, I made it over to their house it was evening time. Since there wasn't anything to do we watched the Bodyguard with Whitney Houston in it. I love Whitney and Ethan knew this. There was a certain part in the movie where she said, but I can't f*** you. He knew I was going to repeat the movie word for word. He wanted to see if I was up for sex that night so he played the movie. We had our own little codes and everything to let each other know when we wanted to have sex. After everyone went to sleep he wanted to have sex I was nervous, because we didn't have protection. I did it anyway, because I really wanted it. During the day I spent time with his mom. Since we had fun his mom asked me to come the next weekend, so I did. We didn't do anything that weekend, because he got sick. While everyone was sleeping I sat up with him and took care of him. The next morning since he wasn't feeling better his father and some other man came and took him and his mom to the hospital. They wrapped him in a sheet and carried him to the car. He looked like a fragile baby. His father "excuse my language" scared the shit out of me the way he was staring at me. He had a mental breakdown when his brother was killed. When they made it back from the hospital they told me he had pneumonia. That night I sat up and watched him, because he was still running a fever. By the morning he was feeling a lot better and again he thanked me for being there for him before I went home *that afternoon. When he got better he came over my house to meet up with my brother the next weekend to meet some girls. I got mad and we got into a huge argument. He didn't come over for awhile and I didn't go to his house for awhile. It was the middle of the school year when he called me and talked me into coming to his house for the weekend saying his mom wanted me over there. 1993 had come and it was spring break we decided to make up. We were doing well not arguing until he moved. The apartments they moved to, they knew many people and some were girls. His brother would tell me he was talking to other girls and of course when I asked he denied it. Until this particular girl came and he told me he wanted to break up. We got into it a huge argument and I went home. I didn't go around for months. As summer was coming near he talked me into coming to his house. He said he was sorry and he made a mistake. That night I wanted him to use a condom and he said he didn't have one, even though he didn't we did our normal routine when everyone went to sleep. I really started getting paranoid about getting pregnant. I was dumb even though I was scared of getting pregnant I had unprotected sex anyway.*

Chapter Three

*I started going back over to his house on the weekends. While I was there
Ethan was outside riding a bike with Garrett and some neighborhood kids. I
was upstairs watching TV, when I heard him scream. His mom and my uncle
were outside watching them, so when I made it downstairs they were picking
him up off the ground. He had fallen off the bike and hurt himself. Since he
was having a hard time standing up they called my dad to come and take him
to the hospital. They carried him upstairs and took him to his mom's bedroom
to watch TV, until my dad came. When I was about to leave the room he asked
me to stay with him until my dad came. It took a couple of hours for him to
come and in that time we made out. I thought he could not be hurt. When my
dad came and took him to the hospital I stayed at his house. When they made
it back, he had chipped a piece of his hipbone, so he couldn't do anything for
awhile. When he finally healed and I went over to his house, we went back to
our normal routine when everyone went to sleep. We both came to an agreement
to just be sex partners, because being in a relationship was to exhausting. One
weekend I went over there he had new girlfriend named Sara. One day he got
into an argument with her, because she was on him about school. He came to
me that night thinking we were going have sex. We didn't do anything, because
I couldn't do that to Sara. She was a sweet girl and I wouldn't want anyone
to do that to me. She always came to me to talk about him. The first time she
came to talk to me about him it was awkward for me. She asked me where I
was going and I told her to get something to eat and she followed me. While
we were talking I tried to explain to her why Ethan was the way he was. After
we talked she forgave him and they made up. I never said anything bad about
him to her. He didn't like the fact that she liked me. He always thought I was
telling her bad things about him, so he would watch us when we were together.
Ethan pissed Garrett off by kicking him out of the room so he and Sara could
have sex one night. He got mad and said he was going to tell. I was outside
downstairs going to the store with another girl when I saw Garrett running
and crying. I ran upstairs to him because, I thought he was hurt. He told me*

what was happening and I just looked at him with this crazy look on my face. When their mom came outside her friend's house were talking, and he told her Sara and Ethan were in the bedroom having sex. She told us to come with her. If I was smart I would've went back downstairs and went to the store. When we made it in the house I stayed in the living room. She busted in the room and said I gotcha and they jumped up. Ethan got mad and punched a hole in the wall. Even though she fussed at them, it served no purpose she didn't tell the girl's parents and she still left them alone together. Then when it was all said and done Ethan's mom said I was the one who told. I had no reason to tell, because that could have easily been me with him and got caught. After that I didn't go over there as much. Sara was in love with him too. She wanted him to accomplish things just like me. I started to realize then he did not love me the way he claimed he did. The things that he was doing with her he never did with me. When his mom called me to come over I did. When I got over there Ethan was in the room crying listening to Babyface. I asked him what was wrong he said Sara was going to move and they had to breakup. So it seems as summer came closer to ending it seemed like they did too. I tried to comfort him in his sadden state. When I did he thought it was a sex invite. (it wasn't) I understood how he felt, because I felt that way about him. We did not have sex, because I could not sell myself short. To be his rebound girl. Well they didn't completely break up after she moved they talked on the phone and she came to visit every now and then. I don't know if he wanted it or she wanted it more whichever way their relationship ended. They were together maybe a year. That was longest he had ever messed with someone outside me at that time.

Chapter Four

The summer of 1994 came and I was ready to relax and have fun. That was my last summer of freedom little did I know. A week before summer vacation Ethan's mom called and wanted to make sure I was coming over when summer started. When I made it there I had another surprise he had started dating another girl in the apartments. It did not last that long. She saw him for who he was. It started out simple my grandmother was staying at their house for a little while. She and I were very close. I spent my days and nights with her. I used to just sit and talk with her all night and day. She would tell the most interesting stories. Some were real and the others she just wanted to scare the heck out of us kids. While I was staying there for the summer one of my best friends' stepfather kicked her out of the house. Her name was Tonya; she came to me to help her out. I did of course, because I always looked out for her. I asked Ethan's mother could she stay there with me until we found her mom she said yes. The summer was great so far, because we were having a lot of fun. Then Ethan's mom had an asthma attack. He was upset about it and wanted to stay with her. She wouldn't let him. Since he was upset and my grandmother went to spend a couple of weeks at my aunt Terri's house, I told him I would stay with her. She ended up having to stay a week in the hospital. I had no clothes to bath, any toothbrush or comb to brush my teeth or comb my hair. While I was at the hospital with his mom she made sure I ate and we would just sit and talk when she wasn't talking to her visitors. When he came to the hospital to visit his mom we would run around the hospital and make out on the elevators. One day while his mom and I were watching TV her mom had called. Her heart rate sky rocketed. The heart machine was going crazy. She was crying. I didn't know she hadn't talked to her mother in years. They stopped talking because, of some family dispute. I was glad her mother had called her, which is the happiest I had ever seen her. While I was at the hospital my grandmother decided she wanted to go home for awhile. I went with her, because I loved her so much and didn't want her to be at home by herself. We made it to her house in Coupland and it was very quiet. She lived in the part of the apartments where elderly people lived. The first night was kind of scary, because she was very sick. I had always had this big fear when we were sleeping she would die. So I sat up all night and didn't move. When she woke up I was very happy. She wasn't feeling well the next day but she never told me. I guess her sugar was up, she was a diabetic, and she was having a hard time seeing that day. I didn't know what to do, but to call my aunt Terri and she told me she was on her way. When she came she took us to the hospital in the city to get my grandmother checked out. They said her sugar was too high. After they got her sugar down and released her, my aunt took her home with her and I went back over to Ethan's house, because my friend was still over there. As soon as I made it through the door Garrett started telling me that Ethan was messing around with Tonya undercover while they were watching TV. When I asked him about it he denied it. We argued for a while, and then he once again convinced me his brother was lying. I left the subject alone, because she left the following day. Her mom that abandoned her came and got her. Then one of Ethan's friends needed a place to stay. Holland moved in. When I saw him I told Ethan we went to the same school. I did not know Holland like me every since 6th grade. Ethan thought it was funny, because Holland was obese. He used to make jokes about it and would tell Holland I liked him too. When Holland moved in Ethan started gambling. During the day time Ethan would be with his friends and I would be in the house. Holland came in the house where I was one day. He pulled out all this money and told me, he would buy me anything I wanted. I told him I couldn't take anything from him, because I didn't like him enough to take money and gifts from him. When I told Ethan about the situation he told me I was crazy I should have used him. I told him that is not who I am. He looked at me like I was crazy and went back outside with his friends. I just kept putting up with Ethan teasing me about Holland, because Holland was not his only friend who came on to me. Another one of his friends was a boy named Marcus. Ethan was telling Marcus about our sex life while they were alone. After he would leave Marcus alone with me, he would come on to me. He would say when you are going to let me have a chance with you; Ethan said you're the best sex partner he has ever had. I asked him what was he talking about and he would say you know he doesn't deserve you. He is very sorry, he's just using you. I didn't believe what he was saying to me, because sometimes men say stuff to women to get into their pants. I didn't tell Ethan, Marcus came on to me, because I knew it would break his heart they were best friends. Plus I loved him too much to even consider messing with Marcus. About a week later Ethan found out Holland wanted to have sex with me and date me and it turned out it wasn't just a crush. From that day on when I was there alone, he would tell Holland to come outside with him and his friends so they could shoot dice. Not long after that my uncle told Holland, he had to leave. He never told him why. Holland was too heavy and he began to break *the furniture in the house. After Holland left we started dating again. Ethan and I would have sex at night and during the day act like we could not stand each other. While I was there my uncle and his mom had a lot of company. This certain guy he was a pervert. He knew I was a kid, but he still tried to have sex with me. To solve this problem I made sure when he was there I was never alone until one day he didn't come over anymore. Ethan's sister Carrie came over and asked did we want to spend the weekend at her house. We said yes, because their mom's friend came into town with her boyfriend to spend the weekend. It was going to be too crowded and they were on drugs so I didn't want to be there. When we made it to his sister's house I called my friends Carla and Tonya to let them know I was in the apartments next to our apartments going swimming. They came and we were having a great time in the pool. My best friend Carla's brother liked me. He came too. We were play dunking each other in the water. I liked him as friend only, but Ethan didn't like the fact I was playing with another boy that he knew definitely liked me. He thought I actually liked Sonny, so he got jealous and started flirting with Tonya, the same one that stayed at his house with me. BIG MISTAKE! I told him I got something for him and got out of the pool. He knew I was angry so he ran after me trying to explain. When I made it in his sister's house I grabbed a broom and started hitting him with it. He was laughing; he stopped when I grabbed a knife. He took off running I began chasing him. My best friend Carla saw us and told her brother Sonny to go and get my dad. I chased him around the apartments, when he got to a certain spot I stopped and threw the knife. If he hadn't turned the corner it would have stabbed him in the leg. My dad caught me and picked me up; he asked him what he did to make me so mad. I lied and a said he called me a b****. My dad cussed him out and told him he knew I had a temper and to leave me alone. After my dad left we got back into the pool and I ignored him. I lied, because no one except my two friends and his brother knew we were messing around. When we went in the house to lay down and go to sleep he told me, he just did what he did, because he got jealous Sonny was touching all over me. We went back to his house my brother came over his house to get him to go and mess with some girls. We argued for awhile after my brother went back down to meet one of the girls. While we were arguing we both were crying. He told me if he didn't go my brother would know something was up. I didn't like it, but I said ok you have a point. He then kissed me on the cheek and left. The following week summer school started for him. Every morning before he left he would kiss me on my cheek and whisper I love you. He thought I was sleep, but I wasn't. We began making all these crazy plans and dreams that when I graduate from school I was going to move out of state for college and he would go with me. We began to get even closer than before. We would argue still, but only to have sex later. When he finished summer school I had to start basketball practice. Summer came closer to ending. So we* *made the best of it and spent every moment we could with each other when no one was around. Then one night he told me after we had sex and was holding each other and talking, he was going to sell drugs. I asked him why. He said he was tired of people making fun of him and his brother. He was tired of not having anything. We both started crying and I begged him not to start selling drugs. On the last day I was to be there before school started we got into an argument. I can't remember why. I went to my sister Marnie's house in the neighboring apartments, to tell her I was getting ready to go home. I wanted to thank her for making sure I was taken care of that summer. Somehow I missed Ethan when I was walking back to his house, because he was walking to my sister's house looking for me and I didn't see him. When I went back to my sister's apartments my cousin Ronald was coming out of my sister's apartment and he said Ethan was looking for me. Then he just flat out said he likes you. I don't care what nobody says he likes you. I started laughing and told him he was crazy. I left and went back to my uncle's house and Ethan was in the house alone. He told me he was sorry and he loved me. We hurried up and had sex before anyone came in the house, afterwards I went home. When school started I was busy, so I wasn't able to go over there for the first few weekends. When I did make it over there one weekend after my basketball game Garrett runs up to me and says Ethan's started selling dope. When Ethan saw me he began walking towards me with a smile on his face, but I wasn't smiling I fussed at him for selling drugs and he got angry at me. We argued, but we made up that night. I went home that Sunday; before I left he told me he wanted to have a baby by me. He said he wanted a baby by the time he turned 16 and he wanted the first one to be by me. I told him you must be crazy. I don't want any kids you better find someone else. He was serious.*

Chapter Five

When I went over there the next time it was the night of my birthday, we had sex and he told me he didn't release himself in me. I missed my period for a few months. It was really hard to tell if I was pregnant, because my periods were irregular. After we had sex one day I told him I might be pregnant. His first response was is it mine. So we started arguing. A good thing we started to get dressed before arguing, because his mom came in the house. When his mom came in I told him, how would you like it if I tell your mom I may have a missed period, because I might be pregnant by you. He knew I wasn't going to do it so he called my bluff and said do it. I knew he wanted me to tell his mom he might be a dad. I looked at him with this evil look and said never mind. I wasn't going to give him that satisfaction. He must have sensed how scared I was so he hugged me and said he was sorry. We started trying to figure out what we were going to tell everyone about me might being pregnant. I came up with the idea that I would say that I got raped on the way home from basketball practice and we both came up with giving it up for adoption if I was. See we were afraid of what would happen to us if our families found out the truth. It wasn't easy just going up to my parents and saying I'm pregnant by Ethan. Not only was that the problem, the men in my family were protective of the females. We both knew it wouldn't be a good situation for either of us. With my dad being kind of crazy. He would have beat the crap out me and tried to kill Ethan. He was very protective over me when it came to boys, because I am his youngest daughter. According to him I wasn't suppose to start dating until I turned eighteen years old. My dad didn't mind going to jail or prison behind a boy or man messing with me. Heck he spent most of his and my life in prison, so he wouldn't have minded hurting Ethan if he found out who I might really be pregnant by. There were also other factors, why we felt we had to lie about my pregnancy. I didn't want anyone to know I might be pregnant by Ethan; I didn't want my mom to be hurt if she knew the truth. Instead of us telling the rape story, we just kept playing as if nothing was wrong. He went to school, kept selling drugs, and gambling. I went to school and played basketball. After time went on a little more my stomach started getting hard. I knew definitely then I was pregnant. When I realized this I became more afraid and started doing desperate things. The things that were going through my mind were things like if I don't say anything about it I could cause myself to miscarriage. Before anyone found out and if this happened I wouldn't have to tell everyone what I was doing and I wouldn't be a disappointment to anyone. I also would not have to worry about what my dad would do to Ethan and me. Plus if I miscarried I wouldn't have to lie on a innocent person or better I wouldn't have to lie to my family at all. On some days I pretended I wasn't pregnant, that all this was a dream. I never thought about it until now, but one of my biggest fears was that I didn't want to be a disappointment to anyone. Everyone expected more out of me. I was the quiet one, the one who took school serious and going somewhere with my life. At first I wasn't going to say what I did to try and make myself miscarry, but today I was watching the news and a 19 year old girl let her baby drown in the toilet, then threw it away.(I never got to see the outcome of the situation and why she did it.) This lady on the Nancy Grace show was talking about the girl. All I can tell this woman is you can't judge that girl for what she did. It was wrong. You don't know what it is like to be in that situation. I was in that situation myself and believe me all kinds things go through your head. You get this kind of fear in you that you can't explain. Some young girls are lucky they have parents they can go talk to, parents that are going to except the baby and help them raise the baby, or they have someone they can trust, without telling and getting them in trouble, but some are not so lucky. Their parents probably beat them for it, disown them for it and they have no one to tell them no matter what you can come to me and talk to me and I'll do whatever I can to help you. Some kids are probably afraid that the organizations that are broadcasted will tell their parents what's going on. So by the time they get the courage to do something about the situation it is too late to get an abortion. Where I'm from you get a simple commercial saying if you are pregnant call and get help. At the time I got pregnant there wasn't even that. The important thing about sending a message like that to a teenager you have to tell them more than that in a commercial. Don't get me wrong some are going to call, but imagine how many would call if that commercial list all the things that they can help you with and if they have to let their parents know what was going on. You do have some parents that would act like it's ok they'll work it out somehow and as soon as no one is no longer mediating between them, they would beat or mistreat their child and let the kid know exactly how they really feel about them, the baby the whole entire situation. So I'm asking people before they judge a kid for what their actions in a situation like this, think about what kind of situation they come from. Some girls get pregnant to have someone to love them, because of the broken home they come from. I know the whole thing could be avoided if they just didn't have sex, well face reality as long as an adult tells a kid not to do it they're going to do it. So the best thing people can do is talk to their kids about it, let them know all the consequences that come with those little moments of pleasure. Don't wait until the kid is thirteen, fourteen, fifteen, and try to sit down and talk to them. You see by that time they have talked to other kids and the kids are giving them the wrong information. At least you can get a chance to teach them the importance of protection, before a kid their age having sex or pretending to have sex convince them it's better without protection or to have sex in the first place. Just think if the parents weren't afraid to talk to their kids at a really young age how many teen pregnancies will go down, the S.T.D.'s, the A.I.D.'s. I'm not saying tell your kids it is ok to have sex. Start as early as they start questioning you about their body. School can only teach and show so much. So you as a parent have to pay attention and talk to your kid no matter how embarrassing it is to you or them. That story today on the news just made me want to let everyone know before they judge the girl see what kind of situation she was in. She may be very regretful about what she did to her baby, but probably felt she had no other choice. I'm upset that an innocent child lost its life, probably over something that was very simple to fix, but I'm not god to judge her. Girls I'm not giving you any excuses to kill your babies. I want you to remember you wanted to be an adult when you were having sex, go a step further and except the consequences and responsibilities that comes with it before killing the baby. If you don't want to keep it just give it up for adoption and now they have it where you can just drop the baby off at the fire station, hospital, or police station with no questions asked. If you choose to keep it though there will be some tough times that lay ahead god will never let you fail if you put your heart and soul into whatever you are trying to do and do not forget to always have faith. No matter what you decide to either keep your baby or give it up for adoption. Sorry I got thrown off of track, but this is what I did out of desperation. I would play just like everyone else, I played basketball until I started to show, I had people stand in my stomach, I even punched my stomach every time the baby would move. While I was doing all these things I felt like those were my only options, but they weren't and every time I think about the things I did my heart aches and I hope that one day my baby would forgive me for those things that I did. Even though I did all these things I never miscarried. All I can think of is god wanted my baby to born. Back to the story. Something that I didn't want to see came to light. Tonya was trying to date Ethan. He kept telling me she wasn't my friend and we would argue about it. I would say yes she is and he would say no she isn't. He would never tell me why he said these things to me. Until one day I told him I didn't want to hear what he was saying to me. He then told me watch you are going see. We ended up breaking up over the whole situation. I wasn't in the mood to see him the following weekend, but as usual his mom called and told me she wanted me to *come over. Since I couldn't tell her the truth I went. When I made it over there Tonya was there. I asked her why was she there. She lied to me of course about wanting to see me. I didn't pay any attention to how she would know I was coming to his house. (She was there for him.) He walked up and yelled hey baby I looked around like who he is talking to. When I looked around it was just her and me. I knew he wasn't yelling at me, because we broke up and our relationship was a secret. I asked her what the heck he is talking about. She got nervous and began to laugh and said uh he asked me to be his girlfriend and I said what did you say she said I told him maybe. I cussed her out and told her to get the F*** out of my face. A couple of years before when I first started talking to her as friend she saw him. I told her then you can't have him he is with me. Then I asked her if we were to break up would you ever try to date him. Her answer of course was no you are my best friend I would never date him or anybody you like, a lie! I did not want to be around her or see her again. He came to me that night and we talked. At the time I couldn't be mad about the situation, because he tried to tell me about her for months. A few weeks later I got the flu I was throwing up and had a fever so I couldn't go over to his house. When his mom called I let her know I was sick and couldn't make it that weekend. My mom had given me some medicine before she went to work. I was in a deep sleep and I felt someone staring at me it was Ethan. When he found out that I was sick and wasn't coming he came to me. Since he was there my brother wanted him to go meet some girls with him. This time he didn't go. I was lying on the living room couch he asked me to walk to the park in the apartments. Even though I was sicker than a dog and weak I went. When we made it there I sat on the slide then he stood in front of me. Then it happened the moment I imagined every since I knew him. He asked me to marry him. My heart was screaming yes, but my mouth said no. He started crying and begging me to marry him, I kept saying no. I told him we were too young. His response was we could get his father to sign some papers for us to get married like his sister, because we were just fifteen. I told him no, because I didn't want him to resent me and the baby. I didn't want him later on in life to say if he hadn't gotten me pregnant and married me he could have done something with his life. I also didn't want my baby to grow up in an environment filled with drugs and the police. After I kept telling him no he asked me were we still on for the plans we made when I graduate high school. I said yes. He took care of me that weekend. We kind of grew apart a little after that. I did not go over his house as much. I used basketball practice as an excuse. Since I pulled back from him he started dating someone else. When I did go over there it wasn't to spend the weekend. I went to keep him informed about the baby. He would always tell me don't have my baby call another man daddy. Even if he hadn't said that I would only allow that for a very special person to my child if I'm married. I believe even though you have a bad parent that's your parent and that's who* *you should call mom and dad. If you decide to call your stepparent mom or dad they have to be very special. One of the things that stick in my mind is those days when I went over there, is how he would play with the baby while it was in my stomach. He would make it move and kick like it couldn't wait to hear his voice and feel his touch. As I got bigger, I barely went over there.*

Chapter Six

I moved in with my aunt Terri after my dad and I had this huge fight. My dad was an alcoholic and on drugs, he came in one night and decided he wanted to talk bad about my sisters and I wasn't in the mood to hear it, because it was 2 in the morning. I'm glad something told me to duck after I said it, because if I hadn't my entire jaw would have been broken. He swung so hard he almost fell. I jumped up and ran across the couch and jumped over the arm of the couch. (By this time, I was 6 months pregnant.) I ran to the kitchen and grabbed the biggest knife in the house. He came after me. I started swinging the knife, as I was swinging the knife my mom came into the house from work. She stood in the way. He swung my mom up against the wall, so I went after him again with the knife. She hurried and stood in the middle again and he swung her up against the wall again. So I swung even harder this time. One more time she stood in the middle and he threw her harder and she was knocked out and this time I started stabbing at him hard and fast. If he hadn't fallen between the kitchen table and the freezer I would have stabbed him in his heart. I ran to get my oldest brother David so he could call the cops. That night I had that fight with my dad it change my attitude and my heart towards him. I was told two very painful things that night one was by my dad. He said I was a whore and by the time I turned 20 I would have 5 kids. The second one was by a police officer; he said since my father abused my brother Derek and me we were going to abuse and treats our kids the same way. My brother and I said at the same time you're a damn lie! Neither one of them knew that I was pregnant at the time they told me this. I hope you can kind of see a little why I chose to keep my pregnancy a secret. That night I decided I could never live in the same house with my dad ever again. At that rate either he or I was going to end up dead. (The story of my dad is a book in itself.) Since I was too big to go to his house on a regular basis and even though he had a girlfriend Ethan came to my aunt's house to see me. While he was there he would say to me one day we going to have a house like this bigger and better though. I thought it was sweet of him to say. I knew even then he was still living in a fantasy. I just *agreed with him even though I knew this would never be. I was still going to school every day and making good grades despite all this. I had to quit basketball, because I was beginning to get into a lot of arguments with some of the other girls and it was getting hard for me to run and keep up. Summer was getting near again and I was pregnant and miserable. I had to keep my hands rested on my stomach to push my shirt out so no one could tell I was pregnant. It wasn't hard to do, because my stomach was not that big as most women's is when their pregnant. Within the first month of summer Ethan and I got into an argument. I told him I didn't want anything to do with him when I went into labor. A month later, I woke up having pains one morning. I figured I was going into labor. I went and ran a bath of hot water and sat in it to slow the pains. It worked for a couple of hours. I was thinking to have the baby in the tub and then throw it away since my aunt was the only one there and she was sleep she wouldn't' t have known. Then I thought maybe I could just leave it somewhere instead of throwing it away. The last thought won though. Just go wake my aunt up and tell her that I got raped while walking home from basketball practice. When I woke my aunt up she started cussing me out and asking why didn't I say anything sooner I could have gotten an abortion or something and that I could have harmed myself caring the baby at a young age. We went to get my mom. My aunt was explaining everything to my mom. She was in shock She couldn't say anything. When we made it to the hospital they put me in the bed from the wheelchair, when I got transferred from the wheelchair to the bed my stomach showed. It had swollen up because, it was time to have the baby and my aunts only response when she saw my stomach was where the f**** did that come from. My water broke I didn't know you couldn't stop the fluid. I told the nurse I was peeing on myself and I could not stop it and please do not tell anybody. She started laughing at me and said okay dear. I stayed in labor for 8 hours. After I had the baby I told the caseworker I didn't want the baby, I was a baby myself I couldn't raise a baby. That is when my mom finally spoke to me. She said I had eight kids and I didn't give any of mines away neither will you. Then she told the caseworker if she doesn't want her I'll raise her. My aunt even told the caseworker she would take the baby. I was listening to their conversations and I thought well since one of them was going to have her I might as raise her myself. I couldn't bear to tell her I wasn't raising her, because I didn't want take care my responsibility. When I had my daughter my aunt made them give me an AIDS test and a test to see if I had any STDs. After that I asked my mom did she want to help name the baby, she was too hurt to even give me an answer. My cousin Emily, Sister Heather, aunt Terri, and I came up with a name. I wanted to name her after my idol. A couple of hours after I had the baby I received a call from Ethan, he was crying. I asked what was wrong he said my uncle Donovan was over at his sister's house with him when he found out I had a baby. He said my uncle was* *threatening to kill whoever got me pregnant. He was scared for his life. (My uncle drives around with guns in his car, just in case something bad happens.) I told him don't worry I was going to stick to my story that I got raped. I got to give this to him even though I had told him to stay away from us a month earlier he caught the bus to the hospital in the pouring rain in a hail storm to be with us. (Thank you for that you don't know how much respect I have for you for your actions.)When he made it there I was asleep and my brother Derek and sisters Karen and Mary was somewhere roaming the halls. I woke up to him staring at me. I asked him did he want to see his daughter, he said yes. I had to call the nurse to get her, because every time I went to sleep they took her out of the room. My blood pressure was high and they were giving me medicine to get it down and it made me sleep heavy. When the nurse came in with the baby he started crying. He was so happy and all he could say was that he loved us both. My brother and sisters came into the room and asked why he was there. He pretended like he was worried that I got raped. Now that I think back my brother had to sense something, because he made the joke here come Ethan's mother not realizing it was going to upset me a little bit before Ethan got there. I laugh now, because I threw up everywhere like the exorcist and scared the mess out of my brother. He made my blood pressure rise very high and that's why I threw up. My brother and Ethan walked my sisters to the bus stop. While they were gone Ethan's mom actually did come. She had brought his brother and our pastor with her. When it was time for them to leave she told Ethan to lets go also. He begged and pleaded please let me stay with her, Derek, and the baby. She stuck to no. He left his umbrella there. I want to tell my brother thank you and I love very much. From the day I had your niece to the day we left the hospital you stayed by our side as if you were protecting us. Thank you again. I love you big brother. We stayed in there an entire week. I was visited by so many people. When it was time for us to leave the hospital I didn't have any milk, pampers, or clothes for the baby. My mom, aunt Terri, and some family members bought some clothes for her and a car seat. The hospital gave me a month's worth of milk and pampers for her. When I made it home, since I said I got raped no one made any effort to ask me where the daddy was. A day after we got home my aunt wanted me to go to the grocery store with her. I was walking slow, she turned and yelled hurry your slow behind up you walking like your private area is sore. I just stared at her. Then we both burst out laughing, because she forgot I was hurting there. The following week went to my other aunt Dorothy's house, so my grandmother and aunt could see the baby. I will never forget the talk my grandmother had with me that day. She said to me in her serious voice you know the first one is always a mistake. When you go and have two and three kids that's when you know what you're getting into. Promise me this I said yes ma'am and then she said again promise me this you won't be like everyone else having all these kids and not do something* *with your life. I said yes ma'am, and then she finished by saying after you do something with yourself then you have more. I kept my promise so far Maw Maw. When my grandmother told me that I did the first adult thing I was supposed to do. I was 16 and my baby was 3 months old I took part of the $168.00 the government was giving me for welfare and put us both in life insurance (without anyone telling me to). The following weekend we went to Ethan's to visit my uncle Larry. When we got there Ethan was there, but Ethan was drunk. He kept staring at me and the baby and talking stupid. My heart was beating so fast and hard like someone was beating it with drum sticks; I thought he was going to tell the truth. His sister didn't want him to hold her baby, because he was drunk. He started calling her out of her name and saying I don't need to touch your baby I got my own baby she look way better than your baby and she is a few weeks old. She started laughing at him and telling him you are just drunk, you do not have a baby. He said, "yes I do." I thought for sure everyone caught on to what he was saying. My daughter was a few feet away from him in her car seat. Thank god no one did. That is when I realized he was starting to drink. Later during the week I needed to go find some clothes for the baby in the shopping center by his house and I could talk to him also. My uncle Phillip dropped my brother and me off over there and as soon as we walked into the house everyone wanted to hold and see the baby. My crazy brother started making jokes saying is your hands clean. Garrett is the first one to grab the baby from me. He thought I didn't see him looking at me, then the baby, then his brother, and then the baby. Ethan was afraid to hold the baby while everyone was there, scared they would pay attention to the same features they had. When I got Ethan to himself I cussed him out about how he almost let everyone know the truth the previous weekend. He told me he didn't care so I left, because I was mad. I left my brother and the baby over there with Ethan and his family while I went to the shopping center. I finished shopping and was on my way back to Ethan's house, then here comes my brother marching with the baby mad ready to go home. I don't know why they were about to fight, but my brother was ready to kill Ethan. He kept saying his a** better be glad I was holding my niece. Later that day Ethan called me and told me that my brother kept saying he better be glad he was holding his niece and that he wanted to say man that's my daughter. I knew him not being able to tell people that was his daughter was beginning to take its toll in him. For the rest of the summer I saw him on rare occasions. Even though I rarely saw him I hung around his sister whenever I got the chance, so he could get closer to her in some way. Instead of him taking advantage of this he chose to go and sell drugs and be with different girls.*

Chapter Seven

School came, but my doctor did not release me to go back to school on time. I had to wait a month later. When I did go back I saw Carla, she didn't believe me during the summer when I told her I had a baby. When I put the baby on the phone she said, "girl you can make those baby noises good, quit playing." I took her to my mom's house where the baby was staying until I got out of school. When she saw my baby she said, " you did have a baby, she looks just like you know who. I said I know. I had to fill her in the story I told before she announced it to the world who the daddy was. She is a true friend she kept my secret as long as it was a secret. I think 1994 thru 1995 is time period that I can't forget. I got pregnant on my birthday and O.J. got acquitted on a double murder charge. (I am not saying that is a good or bad thing.) I remember that day O.J. got acquitted. Everyone was so quiet. You could hear a pin drop throughout the whole school. Just before the bell rang to end the period the jury read not guilty. All at once you could hear cheers and screaming and see people crying. Some were crying for the two people who didn't get justice for their murders and some, because a black man finally got off on a murder charge for somebody white murder. I couldn't believe how some of the kids were acting you would have thought they were kin to or knew the victims and O.J.. It really didn't make a difference to me, because I didn't know any of them, plus I had my own problems to worry about. I felt sorry for the kids though their mom wouldn't be there to take part of any of the major events in their lives and even the small things kids cry to their mother about. A few days after that my baby said her first word it was mama. When the counselor and everyone found out that I missed school, because I had a daughter they made me take classes in taking care of a child and home economics. The teacher let everyone know I had a child. At that time I was the only one in that class with a baby. Word got around school fast that I had a baby. Kids were asking all kinds of questions and making the comments that who would have thought I was the type to end up with a baby. It also brought perverted boys into my face. They would say I was sneaking out of windows. One even came on to me after saying he always *thought I was a good girl. I didn't pay anybody any attention, because I loved my baby and nothing could ever make me ashamed I had her. The first year back at school was tough at first. My mom saw how stressed I was and told me whenever I wanted to hang out like a kid my age she would babysit. I think she said this so I wouldn't resent the baby. I can't complain I had plenty of help babysitting. On the weekends and while I was at school my mom, and aunt Terri would babysit, and on Fridays when I wanted to go to the movies my brother Derek did. When it was too cold out to take my baby to my mom's my aunt babysat while I was in school. I want to say thank you to all of them. My aunt worked late at night and my mom also, so even when they were tired they helped me. I decided that year I was going to do whatever it took to get out of school early. The two reasons I felt this way. I knew my grandmother was getting sicker. I wanted at least one of my grandmothers to see me graduate. She was the last one I had. I would tell her you have to stick around long enough to see me graduate and she would tell me she would. Secondly I was starting to feel like I wanted to drop out. So I went to the counselor and he helped me make a plan out. I began to take some of the classes that I needed to graduate early. My grandmother helped me out a lot she would encourage me when we was visiting with her. She would constantly say I am proud of you. This meant the world to me I knew she meant every word she said to me.*

Chapter Eight

Eventually Ethan and my brother Derek started talking again. He and my brother was hanging out. I did not know my brother was at his house. I called over and my brother answered the phone (he pretended like he was Ethan) I told him he needed to come over and take me to the store to buy the baby some clothes. My brother got rude and said, "why would I do that." And I said, "because she's yours." My brother was shocked he said, "it's me, your brother." When he said that my heart sunk. It felt like I had a thousand pound weight on my heart. I pleaded and begged that he didn't tell anyone. He said he wouldn't tell. After he hung up with me he ask Ethan was my baby his, he got nervous and scared my brother told him I'm not going to do anything, but you better handle your business. Sometime later Ethan did come to me and say he can't take not holding his baby when he wanted to, or letting everyone know that she was his. He said she was going to be confused on what to call him. He said, "what she going to say that I'm her cousin or daddy." Then he said maybe if he had another baby it would take the pain away that he couldn't be what he wanted to be to her. I tried to explain to him, he can't replace a baby with another baby all it's going to do is make him want that part that he was already longing for even more. I still tried to hang around his sister, so he could get to know the baby and so he could hold her whenever he wanted. One of those nights he and Marcus asked me and Carla to go with them on a run and we agreed to go. First he took us to these apartments. This girl named Melissa he was dating was there, he told me to switch seats with Marcus, because I was up front at first with him, so she wouldn't get jealous. They got into an argument I was ready to go back home when this happened. Our next stop was going to be some drug spot (that I found out later); while we were riding he started telling me how much he missed me and loved me (we hadn't been intimate for over a year). I have to admit I was falling for him all over again at that moment. When we made it there all four of us went to this back bedroom in this apartment after he sold the drugs to this woman. She went to another apartment and left us there. He didn't see me looking at *him signaling to Marcus to go downstairs. When his friend started talking my friend into going with him I knew what he had planned. He asked me to have sex with him, he said if I loved him I would do it and I told him if he loved me he wouldn't have me have sex in a crack house. I could tell he was frustrated, but he said ok and then we left. The next weekend I was at Ethan's sister house again he asked me to ride with him and Marcus to sell some drugs, I said yes to talk to him. He sent Marcus upstairs to see if everything was ok while he was gone I told Ethan that I wanted him alive and out of jail so he could be there for our daughter. Marcus came back and then he went upstairs while he was gone Marcus came on to me again saying he doesn't deserve me and he wanted to have sex with me, because Ethan was bragging on our sex life again. I made sure I stayed busy with my grandmother, my baby, and school than to worry about my problems with Ethan. The doctors told us that only ten percent of my grandmother heart was working, so I wanted my daughter to spend as much time as she could to get know her. Another good thing about me having a baby early is that one of my grandmothers got see and spend time with her. She enjoyed my grandmothers company. The school year was coming to an end. All the kids were going to the end of year dances and parties I was at home with my baby. It was ok with me, because I didn't really like those kinds of activities. Even though I was busy with school, my baby, and grandmother I made sure that I kept him and his family involved in her first words, the first time she went to the potty, when she started crawling, and when she first started walking. No one in his family was really interested when I called them and let them know what was going on. I would tell my friends watch when the truth comes out about how she is her granddaughter and her niece instead of just my uncle Larry's niece their attitude is going to change. I told them they were going to say that it is different. The way I feel is in this situation is if you love my uncle and you say that you love us shouldn't you care about what is going on with us especially if we were so close? I left the situation alone after I told my friend's how I felt.*

Chapter Nine

I began to realize just a little bit more god had planned for my daughter to come into this world, when she was 7 months and very fussy. You know how every year they show Martin Luther King Jr.'s I have a dream speech on TV. She understood it. One day I was doing laundry and she was screaming and crying. I fed her, changed her diaper, and even burped her, but she wouldn't stop crying. I sat her in front of the TV, while he was talking, she stopped crying and began to listen to it. She was so focused, while he was TV. Saying his speech her eyes never left the TV. You know that is a long speech. I wanted to make sure my mind wasn't playing tricks on me. I began to mess with her like I was always do and normally she would play back, but not this time. She didn't want me to pick her up or anything. I was so shocked by this that I forgot about doing the laundry and stood behind the couch were she was the whole time. I knew then, that is was something special about her. She loves to mess with me. Like when I put her in her play pen and leave out of the room for a few minutes, when I came back , she would be sitting on the floor in front of the play pen. I figured out after her doing this a few times that she was piling the toys on top of each other and climbing out. At the time she wasn't walking, so I stopped putting her in the playpen, so she wouldn't hurt herself climbing out. When she did start walking at nine months she didn't want me to know. I would put her on one of the couches and go to another room for like a minute and come back she would be standing in front of the other couch. I got hip to her though I pretended like I was going to another room after sitting her on the couch. I went around the corner and began to peek at her as soon as I disappeared she climbed down and ran to the other couch. I was so happy that I ran to her in picked her up and began hugging her. I told her I caught you this time, you could walk all along. She just laughed. I called Ethan and his mom as soon I as I stopped celebrating and called my mom. All Ethan's mom said was that's good let me call you back and he wasn't anywhere to be found. Spring break came and I started hanging back with Ethan's sister trying again to let him get to know his daughter. He was busy with two girls, he was dating, selling drugs, and doing only god *knows what else. I finally caught up to him on the city bus. On my way home from Carla's house. We were talking and he asked me would you ever stick me with child support and I told him if anyone finds out that you are the father and you don't handle your business like a man and take care of her I will. He said that's fair. Luckily when I found out I was pregnant his mom left his social security card lying around and I got the number, just in case it did come to that. I was at Carrie's house and Ethan came to me, he told me that, he was about to have a baby with Melissa I got nervous and scared that when Melissa had the baby it would come out looking like my daughter, because at the time she was the splitting image of her dad. My nerves were so bad that I picked up smoking. I didn't know what to do. Ethan seemed like it didn't worry him anymore about our secret. Summer came again and I was hanging with Carrie this time I left the baby with my mom. I had a headache and was lying on her bed. Ethan came in the room I didn't hear him come in. All of a sudden I felt someone touching me between the legs. I jumped up, and then he asked where is my baby? I told him with my mom. My mother took some time off of work so my daughter spent most of the time with her. He started flirting with me and thought I was going to have sex with him, but I didn't. We talked for a little while and then left out the room. He had a friend in the living room waiting on him. I sat and talked with him, his sister, and his friend for an hour then they went outside. He comes back in a few minutes later and says the boy likes me. I guess he was trying to test me. I told him that I didn't like the boy, which I really didn't. He said just talk to him he needs a friend to talk to, because he has some personal problems so I did. The boy really had a thing for me, but I told him right off I'll talk to you as a friend only. I went home after talking to them for a little while. The next time his sister came and picked me up to go swimming at her house. Ethan and his friend were there again. This time Ethan's friend really hit on me, because he told him that I was just playing hard to get. I told him again I'll talk to you only as a friend. While we were at the pool his friend came and stood between my legs while I was lying back with my head and arms on the edge of the pool. When I felt him there I just got up and moved from him. I guess Ethan got mad, because he hurried up and swimmed to me and said give me a kiss. I asked what? He said again give me a kiss I told him no. He really got mad and started yelling at me yeah you like him. I said no I don't. Mind you, he and I had not been intimate in almost two years. His friend didn't like the fact of how he was talking to me. Then they started arguing. It got so heated that they were about to fight. The only thing that I could think of doing was telling Ethan that I loved him and I didn't want to be with his friend, that he was the only one I wanted to be with. He stopped instantly trying to fight. His friend said f*** both of you and left. Later I did tell his friend that was the only way that I could get him to calm down and that I had been telling him that I just wanted to be his friend.*

Needless to say they stopped being friends. Since Ethan got Melissa pregnant she would be at his sister house with him on a regular basis. He would talk to me and she would get jealous. I don't know what he told her about me, but for some reason she didn't like me. I tried being nice to her and everything else that I could think of. She was the first girl I ever saw him beat. While I was at Carrie's house, they were arguing and my cousin Chloe and I left the house with Garrett to go to the pool. Melissa's brothers and sister was there. Some little boy in the pool threw something and hit their sister. She told her brothers that it was Garrett. We all kept telling them it was the other little boy. They didn't care about what we were saying and began to beat the mess out of him. I tried to get to him, but they kept pushing me back. Since I couldn't get to him Chloe and I ran to go get Ethan and Marcus. Ethan grabbed a shot gun and they ran to the pool. We ran after them and when Melissa's brothers saw the shotgun, they stopped fighting his brother, ran, got in their car, and drove off. Someone called the police and when they came he told me to hold this, they won't check you. I opened my hand and saw that it was drugs. It was too late for me to put it anywhere, because the cops were knocking at the door. So I threw it in a hole that was in the wall. The cops started questioning him about the shotgun people say they saw him with. He told them that he didn't have a gun. When they looked everywhere in the house for it they couldn't find it. He had been smart and took it upstairs to the neighbor's house, because he was dating her also. After they had left he started saying I feel like beating a ho's a** tonight. He kept repeating this. I kept trying to talk to him he said her brothers beat up my brother, so I am going to beat up their sister. I pretended like I had to go to the bathroom. When I stood up, he asked, where is my baby? I told at my mom's house. When I went into the house Chloe and I told Melissa we think it's best she went home, because he was angry and he was going to beat her up, because of her brothers. She told us he isn't going to do s***, because she didn't have anything to do with it. Well as we were going outside he came in said come here let me talk to you in the bedroom. She followed him. Next thing we know we heard her screaming. Carrie and I went in the room he was beating her with a broom. I grabbed his nephew and took him in the living room, because he followed us. Then I ran back into the room and helped his sister pull the broom out of his hands. Then he started beating her. It took us a few minutes to pull them apart. We both grabbed him and while we grabbed him he grabbed her hair. We finally pulled him away from her and he pulled out a patch of her hair. She ran out the room and tried to leave he ran after her and grabbed her keys. She told him to give her keys so she could go. He threw them at her and she told him that she was going to call the police. She did and they came looking for him, but he ran upstairs again to his other girlfriend house. The cops asked where he was. I did not say anything. Marcus lied about not knowing where he was. Melissa came back and said he was probably upstairs. When he heard the cops coming upstairs he just came out. They told Marcus they should arrest him too for lying. While they were arresting him he was making threats on her life. I told him while the cops where locking him in the cuffs stop making threats to her before he be in jail for awhile. Since he was still a juvenile, they took in took a youth facility. This is when I learned he knew how to talk his way out of trouble, when he knew he was guilty. The following Monday he went in front of the judge. His mom asked me to go with them. While he was talking to the judge he said your honor I know what I did was wrong I didn't mean to do it. I was just so angry that her brother beat up my little brother. I grew up without a father and I don't want my baby to go through the same thing. She is pregnant with my child and I love her. Then he went into his childhood problems about how he watched men beat his mom and beat them and how he wants to be a better man than those men. He layered it on so thick even the judge started crying and decided to let him go. After Chloe and I helped her, she told her aunt, she did not like me, that I was a b**** and she thinks that I like Ethan. Well her aunt told my aunt Dorothy. Melissa didn't know that her aunt knew mine. My aunts asked me was my baby Ethan's and why Melissa didn't like me. I told them it wasn't and I don't know why she didn't like me. From that day on every now and then someone would ask me if he was the father and the rumors started. The summer was interesting so far. I spent a lot of my free time on the weekends with Ethan's sister and my friends. She enjoyed my company and I enjoyed hers. She was having some problems with her husband so Carla and I tried to help her out. He was getting tired of Ethan and Garrett coming over to their housing eating up the food and not helping them in anyway. He also was fussing about the house being dirty. So we cleaned her house real good we tried to give her some advice on what to do. It helped her for a little while, but he got angry again about her brothers. We went to their mother's house and to visit her in-laws a lot. During the week I spent most of my time with my daughter and my family. When I did hang out with his sister during the week I made sure we didn't go anywhere dangerous, because my daughter was with me. She would have me help her with her kids. While we were at her house a girl came to visit she was looking for Ethan. I didn't say anything to her, because I didn't know her. I thought she was stuck up, because the way she carried herself. He was gone with Melissa. We were having fun with the upstairs neighbor he was dating when he came home. We let him know she came looking for him. He acted like he didn't care. The following weekend Ethan's mom and my uncle moved in with Carrie. I went into Ethan's bedroom looking for him to give him an update on the baby but he wasn't in there. I saw some little pieces of what looked like broken pieces of soap. I didn't know that it was drugs for sure so I asked his mom what was that. She went into the room and put it on the tip of her tongue. She said it was drugs and took it, because I told her that it wasn't a safe place to have that since kids *were running around house. When Ethan got home I let him know his mom had his drugs. She tasted it to make sure, it was drugs. He asked was I sure, she tasted it. I told him yes, and then he got angry. I didn't know why he got angry. When he went and yelled at her for tasting it and got the stuff back from her. He explained to me she used to be on drugs. He did not want her relapsing. That is when he told me the story about how this man had his mother on drugs and was beating her. He also told me how around this time in his life they used to sleep in a car sometimes. When his mom met my uncle he gave them somewhere to live and helped her get off the drugs. That's why she was so intent on keeping her relationship with my uncle. I was beginning to get some of the picture on why things were the way they were with his family. I was over there even more when my uncle and his mom moved in with his sister. I used to love to hear my uncle Larry argue his points. One day I was hanging over there and the upstairs neighbor that Ethan was dating asked me to spend the night at her house and babysit her son, because she had to go to work the next morning and she didn't have anyone to keep her son. I called home and asked my aunt Terri would it be okay if I could spend the night. She said it was ok, because my uncle was downstairs and my baby was with my mom. Derek told my aunt that I was spending the night there, because Marcus liked me, and he would be staying over there also. She then called backed and cussed me out and told me to go downstairs and stay there. I didn't like Marcus I had no intentions on messing with him at all. I was just doing a favor for the woman. Well later on that day Marcus did come on to me again and asked me to have sex with him. Again saying Ethan was bragging about sex with me. I told him you're crazy I am not going to have sex with you. Your best friend was my first at everything in my life when it comes to a man and I could never do that to him. Then he said your baby is his baby. I told him I did not say that. He then said he already knew no matter what I said. Then he went into the house and Ethan came out. We were standing outside talking. He was asking me about the baby and I told him all that he wanted to know. He then started talking to me about his feelings for me, as we got deeper into the conversation my uncle Phillip drove up with my baby. He told me to get in the car I had to go home, because my mom, my aunt Terri, and my sister Marnie went out of town, because my sister's father had died. Most of the rest of the summer I spent my time with my family. My grandmother was getting sicker. We had fun my daughter would sit in my lap and talk to her and play. So we spent most of our time doing that. Carla asked me to come to her house. I went over there and since she lived in the apartments next to Carrie we went to her house. When I got there Ethan was there with another one of his girlfriends. He was getting his hair braided. I started messing with him hitting him. He said stop I'm not in the mood to play, but I kept hitting him anyway. He said stop again and I kept on playing and hitting him. I stopped after a little while and told him he wasn't fun anymore. Then his girlfriend started to hit him, he told her to stop. She kept on and then the next thing I knew he was up punching her. Then he started dragging her and hitting her saying you can't do what she do. You can't ever do what she does. Then her sister ran back to the back to fight him too and he beat her up. When they left and he came back to finish getting his hair braided I told him I'm going to quit playing with you. You are getting too serious for me. He then said I told her she can't do what you do. I could not say anything. A few weeks later his sister moved. That is also when I slowly stop hanging around his sister. The neighborhood, his sister moved to was not safe. I couldn't picture having my daughter in that kind of environment. So I really started spending time with my grandmother. Every now and then I would still hang with Carrie.*

Chapter Ten

Soon school started back again, so I spent less time with them I was doing fine like always, but this school year was different I was going to graduate no matter what in the 1996 to 1997 school year. My daughter and I spent as much time as we could with my grandmother, because the doctor said she didn't have much longer to live. One afternoon Carrie said she could take my mom, my daughter, and me to the hospital to visit her, since my aunt had to go to work. We sat with my grandmother for awhile and my dad was at my mom's house waiting for her. Well as soon as she drove up in the apartments he started cussing my mom out. I know I should not have said what I said. I told him, you are not going to cuss her out, because she was at the hospital visiting with her mom. She just found out that her mother didn't have much longer to live. You need to shut up and be there for her the same way she was there for you when your mother was sick and dying. Everyone told me that he is my father and I shouldn't be talking to him like that. All he could do is look at me and tell my mom he was sorry. After that day I really started working hard in school. I signed up for night school, so I would make sure to graduate in time enough for her to be there. Time was running out and the hospital had signed my grandmother up for a hospice nurse to come out. At first I thought it was a home nurse, but it wasn't. My aunt Terri explained to me the nurse was there to make it easier for my grandmother to go ahead pass away. My aunt Terri did not want them there. She also did not like the fact the doctors was giving up on my grandmother. When my grandmother made it home she really wasn't the same. It was like she was living in two worlds. She was aware that we were there, but she would call certain family members in our family, people in our family who had pasted away. She was holding strange conversations about the past as if they were the dead relatives. Then all of a sudden she would call them by their names and talk to them about current things. It didn't matter to me though, because she was home and I got a chance to spend even more time with her and so did my daughter. I also was used to it from my childhood. Late at night when my grandmother and I would go to bed I would wake up in the *middle of the night to her talking. I would ask her who she was talking to, because I didn't see anyone, and she would say a person or persons in our family that pasted away. I would get scared and pull the cover over my head and go back to sleep. I never asked her what they would talk about. My daughter had just turned one she was walking and talking real good. I remember it like yesterday. Since my grandmother body was shutting down she really couldn't eat solid foods a lot. So my daughter would walk down the hallway saying Maw Maw, so she could feed her jello She would carry the spoon and the jello herself. Then she would sit in my lap and feed my grandmother her jello. Everyday a nurse from Hospice would come and talk to us and my grandmother. One day she just blatantly told us we need to tell her it's ok for her to pass on and we were going to be okay. My aunt Dorothy went in there right away and told her, but no one else could. I don't know how I got up the strength to do so, but a few days later I did. I told her that, but I didn't mean it. Everyday I would try to make a deal with god to make her better. Telling him I would stop doing this and I will do that. Not long I say maybe a month later she left me. I knew the morning my cousin came in screaming for me to wake up. When I got up everyone ran out the house and left me. I had no car and no way to get there. So I called Carrie to pick me up. When I was on the phone with Ethan's mom, I kept telling her, I know she is gone. She kept saying no she not. When I finally got there I went straight to the room where my grandmother lay still. Then her voice came back to me and said when it is somebody you truly care about and they pass away you will be able to touch them and kiss them good bye. I would say no I wouldn't I'm scared of dead people, but she was right I touched her and held on to her until Carla came and told me to come outside with her and take a walk. Since we knew what she died from we had to wait on the funeral home to come and get her and that took hours. I think we walked for about 3 hours straight. When we made it back the funeral home was there. (Thank you Carla you will always be my sister until the day I die.) I held up better than I thought at the funeral, because we expected her to jump up out her casket to slap my cousin Emily. You see my cousin and her would always get into arguments and she would tell her don't come to my funeral when I die. I'm going to jump up out of my casket and slap the s*** out of you. Of course it never happened. After the funeral is a different story, because I was so angry she was gone that I actually stop believing in god. I tried to make a deal with god; I stopped doing things and began doing others. but it didn't work. The only time I would go to church was for a funeral or wedding past that you couldn't talk to me about god. What made me miss her most was when my daughter would go to the refrigerator and get a cup of jello and a spoon, go to the room, and yell her name. I can't talk much longer, because it is hard to keep the tears back, today made it 14 years she has been gone. After my grandmother past away I really buckled down to be the best person and mother*

I could be. I wanted to keep the promise I made her. I kept going to day and night school. I thought I wasn't going to be able to graduate that school year. I missed some school, because my grandmother past away that fall. I was having a hard time with a babysitter, because my mom had to go back to work and my aunt Terri was complaining about me getting home in time from school to get my daughter for her to go to work on time so something had to give. My other aunt Dorothy stepped in and kept my daughter for me while I was in night school. That way I could walk to her house after I get out of school, to get my baby. My uncle Phillip would pick us up and take us home. I was finally back on track and then my daughter got sick. The last semester I had to go and a week before finals. As you can guess I missed a week of school. The teacher knew I had a baby and that she had gotten sick, but he didn't cut me any slack. I failed my final exam, because I missed that last part he taught it was majority of the test. Algebra 2 was the only class I needed to graduate. I was already having trouble with a babysitter, so I started crying, because I did not know how I would be able to go to summer school. My aunt Terri told me I would keep her. Make sure you come straight home after you get out of school. I kept my promise and she hers. That school year I hung with Carrie rarely. On one of those days I met their cousin Simon. He was in love with me from the first time he saw me. I knew nothing could come out of it. He would take off his shirt to impress me. I didn't allow myself to feel anything, he was Ethan's cousin. Carrie kept trying to get me to talk to him. One day she and her husband asked me why I don't talk to him he really liked me. I told them I couldn't talk to him, because he used to mess with a girl my cousin Ronald used to date. They said that was no reason for me not to talk to him. I just talked to him as a friend. While we were riding to Ethan's mother house Carrie and I were talking. She said, I'd die for you. I asked where that came from. She said I'm just saying I would, and then Simon said he would die for me also. Then she asked Simon would he die for her he said h*** no. Then they started arguing and I was relieved that they did, because I wasn't about to lie and tell either of them that I would die for them. After they stopped arguing, he tells me, he would sell drugs to take care of me and my daughter. I told him he wasn't going to use my daughter and me to say that he was going to sell drugs. If he were going to sell drugs, it would be for him. I told him that I don't want a man that is doing the wrong thing and harming people for their personal gain. He sat back and thought about it. I didn't know that Carrie was telling Ethan about his cousin liking me. Ethan was back with one of his old girlfriends, so I didn't know and understand why he was making comments and coming on to me even when Simon and Carrie was around. It comes to me now, he wanted them to know in some way I was his. He didn't want him trying to date me. Carrie told Ethan she saw me and Simon kissing. When he called me fussing at me I didn't know why he was fussing at me. I was sleep when he kissed me,

I found out about it when he called fussing at me. I was exhausted, because the baby had been sick and fussy all week. I did not have any sleep. When she went to sleep that night I fell asleep too. I didn't feel anything, because I was in a deep sleep. He didn't believe me. I tried to explain to him I would never date his cousin, because we had a baby together and I loved him. One day I caught the bus to Carrie's house Simon was on the bus. He went with me to her house. When we got there Garrett told us Ethan was going to beat him up. I asked why and he said Simon stole Ethan's money. He said he didn't and he wanted to talk to Ethan face to face. So he, Garrett, and I went to Ethan's mom house where Ethan was. When we made it there Ethan was ready to fight. Before Simon could get anything out Ethan jumped him. My uncle Larry grabbed Ethan and he told me to take Simon in the bedroom. When I locked the door. Ethan became angrier. When he left Simon took that time to leave too. I stayed. When Ethan came back I talked to him. He asked me did I like Simon I told him no. I asked him, how did Simon end up stealing his money. He said while he and his girlfriend were in the bed sleep. I told him he needs to sleep with his money in his underwear then he will know who took his money, because no one but his girl will go in his underwear.I think she took his money. If she didn't, maybe he was looking for a reason to fight Simon for kissing me. Needless to say I stopped going around them for a little while.

Chapter Eleven

By the time August came I was excited, because I was about to graduate. I graduated August 26, 1997. That day was one of my greatest milestones in my life. Since my grandmother wasn't there to share it with me, I was glad my daughter, mother, and the rest of my family were there to cheer me on. As I was walking across the stage all I could think was a year early, so far I was keeping my promise to my grandmother. By September 4, 1997 I had a full time job and enrolled in some classes at the community college. I couldn't take many classes, because I had to pay out of my pocket to take classes. My major was pre-med. I was doing great for a year. I had a dilemma, I found out that to be a doctor you had to work on a dead body.(there goes my childhood dream) Ethan's mom asked me to come over her house sometimes still on the weekends since my mom kept my daughter. I finally started going back over there a year after my grandmother past away. He was dating this new girl Holly. I didn't care whether or not he was dating, because I moved on. His mom called me over and decided to leave as soon I got there. She said I need to go on a run right quick you can come with me or you can hang with Holly. I didn't want to do neither, Ethan's mom was going to a place I knew I was going to get in trouble for being there and I really didn't know this girl. I told his mom I was going home. She said, just go with Holly to the doctor and I should be finished by the time she is done. Since no one still knew about my daughter's dad I couldn't come up with a good excuse not to go. When we got there all Holly was doing was talking bad about Ethan's family and him. I wouldn't say anything about them with her I would change the subject a lot. I was glad when the doctor called her name. They told her that she was pregnant. We finally went back to his mom's house. When we got there Holly was pretending like she just really loved their company. She told his mom the news and they were happy. I was just ready to go home; because he was there when we got back and when no one was around he would come on to me. I couldn't do it, because he was dating and she was pregnant with his child. When I told them I was going home Holly offered to take me and asked for my pager number so we could *hang out. I really didn't want to, but I gave it to her anyways. She paged me a lot; she said I was fun to talk to. I became her friend. She was crying and complaining about how Ethan was treating her and I would give her the best advice I could. When I caught him by himself I told him he needed to stop treating her bad, because she was pregnant with his child, he would say that isn't my baby. Even though I found out she was still messing with her ex around the time she got pregnant, I told him he was wrong for what he was doing and he needed to take care of his responsibilities. Then he would ask me what me and my daughter needed I told him we were fine, when I needed his help I would let him know. He told me to let him know whatever we need. I didn't know, when I wasn't around he would tell Holly that I was hanging with her, because I liked him. That wasn't true. I just got caught up in hanging with her, because no one knew who my daughter's father was and I couldn't be mean to someone who had never hurt me. We didn't hang out every weekend, but we hung out enough to become real good friends. She had fallen head over heels in love with him and was letting him just dog her and beat the crap out of her. When she went into labor she called me I didn't want to go. I made up a lot excuses to her for me not to be there, but in the end I ended up going. I ended up going, because she was crying he wasn't there and how much she wanted me to be there with her and her family. He never showed up while I was there I don't know if he even showed up that day. He would make her very angry, because she wasn't working and he was mistreating her and the baby. After she had the baby we weren't hanging out as much as we used to. I went to visit my sister Mary, so happen Ethan and Holly were living in the same apartments. When she saw me they were in the middle of an argument and she turned and walked away crying. I followed her to see if she was okay and my brother Derek stayed and talked to him. She started telling me, he wouldn't give her money to get the baby food and pampers and they were sleeping on a roach infested floor. I had to get back to my brother before he left me and she went back into the house. My brother's girlfriend lived over there too, when she came home he went up there for a few minutes. I sat outside talking to Ethan about his situation. He said f*** her. What does my baby need? What do you need, I told him again we are fine you need to help her get the baby a decent place to live and help her more. Then he kept saying where my baby at, I told him at my moms. After that I didn't see them for some months. I was still working full time. Holly called me and wanted me to hang with her at the mall, I told her okay. I didn't know Ethan was going to be there, I guess when he saw me he got angry and they started arguing. We left the mall together and left him. While we were on the bus she asked me did me and him mess around and is he my daughter's father, because she had heard some rumors. I told her that it is not my place to tell her any of that she needed to talk with him. She said she would and I guess he lied to her, because she didn't ask anymore. Some more* *months went by before I saw her, because I was still juggling work and some of my own problems. I had just about done a year at my job when I quit. I quit, because the owner of the company had died and his kids took over and made going to work miserable. Since I wasn't working I decided to take my daughter with me, when I went to go meet her at the mall this time. When we were on the phone she had told me she stole Ethan's drugs and sold some of them so she could go get her baby some clothes. I told her he was going to be angry and may do something to her. She said she didn't care and wasn't scared of him. I met her at the mall and she bought the kids some shoes. I told her she didn't have to buy any for my daughter, but she did anyways. At this time she was living with a friend and Ethan was living with his mom. He called her at her friend's house and told her to come to his mom's. Since I didn't have anywhere else to go I told her I would go with her when she asked me to. When we got there he was angry, they argued for a while in his mother's bedroom. I heard him tell her give him his drugs she told him she sold them and then he hit her. He hit her while she had the baby in her arms (his mom was standing there in the room the whole time). I ran in there to get the baby, and then covered my daughter ears so she could not hear. She broke free and ran out the house and called the cops. He ran. I was still shocked and when the cops asked me what he had on, I just blurted it out without thinking before I talked. He ended up calling me a couple of days later and asked me why I snitched him out. I was honest I told him I just blurted it out without thinking. Holly was being a trouble maker then and tried to make him mad at me. Mind you all this time he was still trying to get with me behind her back, but I wouldn't do it. I didn't talk to them both for a month. Holly called me and said she got a job and to see if I had found one too. When I told her no she told me to come to her job and apply. Since I had a child to take care of I went. I got hired. We were on the same shift. We hung out with two other people while we worked there one was a man and the other was a woman. She and Ethan were still together, but she got interested in our co-worker. She started ignoring him and everything. I would still see him once in a while. He wanted me to tell him what she was doing and flirting with me at the same time. I never would respond to his advances, because I was friends with her. She worked there about 6 months and in those 6 months we went from the four musketeers to two when it came to lunch. She and the male co-worker would go off for an hour at lunch together. I never would tell Ethan her business, because he was cheating too. When she got fired I wasn't able to talk and hang with her that much, because I was working still, by the time I made it home I was tired. One day she finally called while I was on the city bus. Some kind of argument was going on between her and my cousin Stacy and some other people. I told her I wasn't worried about what my cousin said, because I know I didn't say anything about anyone. When I hung up with her my cousin called. I told her I have no idea what they* *were talking about, because I hadn't hung with Holly in awhile and we rarely talked on the phone since I had to work. Then when I made it home my messy cousin was there she called Holly on a three way call, I didn't know that she had just hung up the phone with her when I walked in. She started talking crazy to me and I argued right back. While both of them were on the phone I repeated everything I said to the both of them while I was on the city bus. I had nothing to hide, because I didn't say anything wrong about anybody. My cousin couldn't say anything else to me, because what Holly told her was a lie and all Holly could say was, but you don't hang with me, you don't talk to me. I kept saying in front of my cousin that is not what I said and tried to tell Holly what I said. Since both just got busted in a lie, she kept interrupting me saying the same thing you don't hang with me, you don't talk to me. So I just hung up the phone and my cousin was looking stupid. My aunt Terri took this time and situation to ask me who my daughter dad was. I thought about it I didn't know what all Holly had told them and then I was also tired it had almost been 3 years I have kept the lie going it was time to tell the truth. I told her who the father was. She made me call my mom and tell her the truth and then she told me to call his mom and tell her. I told her I wasn't telling her anything, she didn't care about what was going on with my daughter. So she called her. She did exactly what I said she would. She got emotional and started saying for three years you kept my grandchild from me, I told her, her son knew and I tried to let her know everything that was going on in her life and invited her to every birthday party. She didn't care when it was just my uncle niece and she never showed up to any birthday party. She started talking crazy to me and I just handed the phone back to my aunt. His mom called him and asked him and then he denied it she called me back and told me what he said. I called him and told him he needs to tell her the truth, because she was hurting. We got into it for a little bit, he told me am I going to be like these other h*** and put the government in our business. I told him you remember me telling you if you weren't handling your business like a man I would. He told me yes he did. He wanted to make sure my aunt knew I went after him first. I said no I didn't, because I thought he was talking about right before I got pregnant and then we hung up. (Now that I know what he meant, yes I did and I wouldn't change a thing. I wouldn't have my baby.) Later everybody was talking about me at every family function. Everywhere I went someone was looking at me and talking about me. Holly got angry when she found out that my daughter belonged to him. She started yelling I asked you, I told her even then, it is not my place to talk to her about that, she needs to discuss that with him. I did let her know that as long as she and I were friends I never slept with him, because I valued our friendship more than that. She never believed me I know I told her the truth, so it didn't bother me. I was putting my child aside for hers to get taken care of. Thanksgiving came and his mom introduced herself to my* *daughter as her grandmother. I am not a racist, before I put this down and my daughter was 2. My daughter looked at her didn't say a word to her; she eased to where I was and tugged at my clothes. I bent down and asked her what was wrong. She said that woman said she is my grandma. I said to her yes she is. Then she said, but she is Mexican. I guess she was looking at the fact they were two different skin colors. I told her, her father was mixed and she just stared at her and said oh. When I told his mom what she said she just started laughing. My aunt Terri made me take a picture of my daughter to Ethan's mom house a few days later, because she felt, since she was the grandma she should have it. While I was there, I let her know he didn't hit me or treat me like the other girls, because she was trying to convince me to start dating him again and he didn't hit girls anymore. He was still with Holly. I didn't communicate with any of them for awhile. One day I got a phone call from his mom telling me that Holly was going out of town and he was going to be at her house and if I wanted to come over. I told her I couldn't come, because I was busy. This went on until my daughter 3rd birthday I called him to see if he was coming to her party. He lied like he was. At midnight that night I walked down to the mailbox and dropped the child support papers in the mailbox, because he didn't show. A couple of months later I get a call from his mom saying someone in their family past away and could I bring my daughter. I told her I would bring her over after the funeral. When we drove up to her house everyone was almost gone except her uncle. As soon as my daughter got out the car he said that is my niece I don't care what no one says that is my niece she looks just like us. His mom agreed with her uncle. I didn't talk to anyone in his family for about four months and then his mom called me talking about him, trying to get me to date him again. I told her I was happy he changed and I met someone that treated me and my daughter well. Man that must of made her angry. We went to child support court a little while later and he had the nerve to ask for a blood test. Even the lady giving the blood test shook her head at him. My guess, she was thinking she looks just like him and he kept telling my daughter it didn't hurt daddy, because she was crying. When we made it home my whole family got angry when my daughter said they poked her finger and I had to explain they did a blood test. My family was angry, because my daughter looked just like him. The next evening I was on a date and his mom called me cussing me out and saying she told him to ask for the blood test. I told her she look more like your family than your daughter's kids. She told me looks don't mean anything. Ethan didn't know the baby was his it could be anybody baby. I then told her he knew that is why he was begging and crying to stay in the hospital with us. She then said he never went to the hospital when I had my baby. I told her yes he did, he left his umbrella, I still have it do you think he would want it back. She got real angry then and started cussing me out worse. I cussed her back out. I told her he was going to have to pay the state back and everything* *that she was saying to me I was going to make her eat every single word. Then my uncle took the phone from her and told me to quit calling his house starting trouble and she called me. I didn't have anything to say to him or his mother anymore. I didn't see them again until the next time we went to court. The judge read out the words to him that you are 99.99% the father. His mom face had dropped, because she told another woman my daughter was her granddaughter. We both took turns on the stand in front of the judge to tell our story. He kept telling the story how he didn't know the baby was his, because he didn't want to have to pay all the back pay, not realizing whether he knew or not he still had to pay the back pay. He got off lucky though, because we were minors when we had her they took those years off. When I got on the stand I told the truth, basically what I'm telling you guys now. We had to get a caseworker for our case, because we couldn't come up with an agreement for visitation. After court his mom started talking to this lawyer that was in the courtroom, thinking they had a good case. When he went into the bathroom his mom and Holly started calling me out of my name. Since I was trying to control my temper, because my daughter was with me I went outside to tell my aunt Terri what was going on. We went back in the lobby and they were there still talking. My daughter tried to throw her shoe at them. The sheriff came over, because she heard us talking. She said don't worry about them, look at them they are trashy and you can tell they aren't going anywhere in life. When she gets older they're going to have to pay for all the things they are saying and doing, and that is going to hurt them more than what they are doing to her and you right now. After that the judge called our names again. They let us know when was the next time we had to go to court. When we went home my family went to their house to approach him and his mother about them calling me out my name, of course they told me that they were going to the store. I didn't find out they went over there until they came back. I went ahead the next day and called me a lawyer too. When I met with him that Monday he told me he would take my case for 2,000 dollars. I didn't know how I was going to come up with the money; I was just a cashier at the grocery store. The dude I called myself dating gave me $800.00 (Don't let this gesture by him fool you about him, again I can write a whole book about him too.) and my aunt Terri went and got a loan for $700.00 and I had $500.00 saved up. After this the caseworker just showed up at my house. She told me I had to do a random drug test, because there were accusations that I was on drugs. I told her to hold on while I ask my aunt Terri to watch my daughter so I can go. As I was walking to my aunt's room she saw the caseworker go into my room to wake up my daughter. My aunt walked into my room and lay in the bed with my daughter so I could leave with the caseworker. The caseworker was insistent to talk to my daughter, but she wouldn't wake up. As soon as my daughter turned her face toward the caseworker she said Ethan lied. I said huh she said she looks just* *like him, there is no way possible he did not know she was his. My aunt told her that is what we have been trying to tell the judge. When we left for me to take the drug test she explained to me whatever we discussed stays between her and me. I didn't know she had already talked to Ethan, his mom, and Holly. I didn't find that out until a few days later when my uncle called and threatened to kill me and my aunt Terri, because Ethan's mom lied like she was hiding in another room and told my uncle I told the woman he did something to her daughter. I tried to tell him I didn't do that and he still cussed me out. I called the caseworker and told her what happened and she said for me not to worry about it, because she was going to handle it. She said his mother was sitting right there the whole entire time when she talked to him and even described her to me. She said she told them the same thing she told me that what was discussed in that meeting was to stay in that meeting. When we went back to court to determine the visitation the caseworker was there. She sought me out and was standing with me until she saw his mom and excused herself. Whatever she said to his mom she left the courthouse. My lawyer was there with me. This time I didn't have to get on the stand. The caseworker was the only one who had to get up on the stand. She told the judge she felt that Ethan needed supervised visitation, because he had all these pending charges and he had yet to go take his drug test and I took mine with no problem. She also suggested that my daughter not be allowed near his mom, because she was the one keeping trouble going between me, Ethan, and the rest of the family. The judge agreed with the caseworker and granted temporary supervised visitation, to give him a chance to change his ways. She asked him did he have a problem with my aunt Terri being the supervisor, because there was no one else and it was free. Before he agreed he told the judge that I sent my family to his house to fight them. I told the judge that I didn't know they were going over there I was told they were going to the grocery store. She told him I don't have control over what other people do if they didn't tell me anything. I was getting frustrated with the whole thing. I was working part-time and taking care of my daughter helping her with her homework. When she began school I knew she was smart, but I didn't realize how smart. I knew she was smart, because she started reading at three. There was no infomercial back then teaching kids to read at an even earlier age. She was doing great in school she was picking things up quickly. The first time Ethan came to visit I had just had surgery. I had a polyp removed and it turned out to be precancerous. He knew I was in the bedroom, so he would make it a point to have to keep going to the bathroom, which is by my bedroom. My daughter didn't want to visit with him so she hid under the bed. My aunt had to go under the bed and get her. He didn't know what to say to her so he talked about me with me her. My daughter climbed in the bed with me after he left and told me he told her things she already knew about me, I told her to be nice he was just trying to talk to her. She told me that he promised to get her some sidewalk chalk shaped like ice cream. I don't know why he done that, because she held him to that promise, he never came through. He made a few more visits after that. He would always find a reason to talk to me alone. When I would go with him, he would flirt. I never gave in to him, because I was dating someone. The next time I saw him was at court he showed up late as usual. The judge and my lawyer were trying to get me to take his parental rights away since he wasn't there. I told them I would rather just keep the supervised visitation, because she may want to get to know him and it would break his heart. Since he wasn't paying the lawyer she asked the judge to be taken off the case. Ethan's mom didn't know that and tried to talk to the lawyer. She told her she wasn't representing her son anymore he needed to learn how to pay his child support and bills. When he made it in there the judge told him I had sole custody and he had supervised visitation permanently. He asked what about his family getting to know his daughter, she told him I suggest you don't piss mommy off then.*

Chapter Twelve

It was now 2000 and my daughter had started school seven months before. She had started Pre-K that year. It was the first time I had to take her to the hospital also. She got bored in the cafeteria and decided to stuff only god knows how many paper towels in her ear one Friday. (She says she was aiming to put 20 whole paper towels in her ear and only made it 15.) She didn't tell me. She told me Sunday, only, because her ear started hurting. When we couldn't get it out by ourselves we took her to the emergency room. They used a syringe with a hose at the end of it to squirt the paper towels out of her ear. My aunt Terri told me you better take that, because you know she is going to do it again. Sure enough she did. That was not the scariest things she had done. While I was in the refrigerator getting milk to fix her a bottle she somehow opened the cabinet door under the kitchen sink and was about to drink some ammonia, I immediately dropped the milk and stuck my finger down her throat to make her throw up just in case she did drink some and then gave her some milk to coat her stomach. The most scary thing was when she was 2 I had sat her in my room to watch TV. She found a penny somewhere and swallowed it. (She says she thought chocolate was inside of it.) I was cleaning the house when she ran to me and her lips were turning purple. I tried the hymleich maneuver, but it didn't work, so I took my finger and stuck it down her throat. I made sure I didn't go straight down in the middle so I wouldn't knock the penny further down and kill her. I went to the side and stuck my finger all the way down her throat and hooked the penny. I slowly brought my finger back up and by time I finished throw up was all over me and the floor. She was crying and screaming. I did not care, because my baby was ok. My daughter and I were doing fine. She kind of hit a rough spot in school. She was a little different from the other kids. She would rather sit and talk with the teacher at recess than play. I tried to get her to play with the other kids, but she wouldn't. By this time I was working full-time for a loan company. Technically that is what it was. The first location they placed me at was supposed to be check cashing, but you can get money if you had some vouchers for a catalog. I picked up on the job quick. I had just gotten used to that place, when one day I was eating lunch and my manager came and said they were shutting down all the check cashing stores. One of the girls at the other store stole a couple of thousand of dollars. The owner was like this if one person steals everyone gets fired. When I was on my way home, I got a phone call from the girl I worked with and she told me to file for unemployed. I never got fired before, so I didn't know I could do that. When I made it home my aunt Terri told me my job had called. I called them back and they told me that if I wanted I could go and work at the main store. She said she liked the way I handled myself and I was a smart girl. I was a little scared about working at that store, because 4 girls got murdered in that building. I needed the job so I could take of my daughter. Needless to say I took it. I had been working in the building about three months when the anniversary of the murders came. A lot of crazy people came out for the anniversary. I was waiting on a customer when a gypsy woman claiming to be psychic was running something up and down the outside wall. After the customer left I stood outside laughing at her, because at first she was at the wrong window, saying she feel their presence. She wasn't the only psychic there, but she was the funniest. Then there were the news crews. I was kind of afraid to close that night, because there were a lot of crazy people hanging out to be on the news. A few days before Valentine's Day Ethan and I went to court. He was flirting with me, Derek and my boyfriend was sitting there too. He didn't know the dude was my boyfriend though. My brother told my boyfriend to sit down and shut up I knew how to handle myself and he was no match for Ethan. When Ethan found out that I was dating this dude he called me while I was at work angry. First thing he asked me was who that man at court with me was. I asked him why he said that he was told by his sister that I was dating the dude. (She saw me getting off the bus one day and followed me to his apartment.) I said he hangs with my brother Derek too, does that mean he is dating him too. I ended up telling him I was dating him and he told me that he didn't expect me to date anyone but him. We got to talking and I told him about how all his friends would try getting me to have sex with them, because he would talk about our sex life. He tried to tell me he never talked about our sex life. I proved my point when I told him everything Marcus said to me. He then accused me of liking it and wanting to do it. I just simply told him how I felt. That my heart belonged to him and so I didn't feel the need to ruin his friendships, because I knew I would never mess with any of them. We hung up after he asked me about my daughter and I told him my brother Derek was babysitting her. A little while later he called my house to speak to my daughter. When I told her who was on the phone, she did not want to speak. I told him she didn't want to talk to him. He said let my baby tell me that. When I handed her the phone she got angry. Whatever he was saying she didn't want to hear it, because all she said was no a couple of times. She then shoved me the phone like it had feces on it. She then stormed out of the room. I immediately asked him what he said to her, because she did those things. He said all he asked was did she want to spend time with him. After that he didn't call.

Chapter Thirteen

I didn't feel the place was hunted until I bought a dog from a co-worker. He brought some puppies with him to get his paycheck. I was sitting at my desk when one of them climbed out the box and came to me. I told him I wanted him. He told me he can give him to me in a couple of weeks. When I went to pick my puppy up he was afraid of being in the back of the store. He used the bathroom nonstop while he was in the store, so I took him outside to the bathroom. As we were going back into the building he ran away and I had to chase him and carry him in the building. Since I had a job I couldn't spend the time I wanted with my daughter. My brother Derek had begun going to church and he wanted me to go. I really didn't want to. I stopped believing in god and felt there was no need to waist my Sundays.(I guess god knew I would need him working in the place I did and the journey I was about to take.) My brother bugged me to the point I said if I go will you stop harassing me about it. The following Sunday we went to church. When I walked through the door I was angry. I really didn't want to be there. The pastor started preaching. At first I was in my own world looking around, but mainly at the floor and then I started listening. When I looked up toward the preacher he was looking at me. The sermon was about when we've completed the job god gave us to do on earth he picks our flower and it is time to go home and live in the land of milk and honey. By the time he finished, he made me feel real bad about the person who I had become. For the last 4 years I was very selfish, I never stopped to think about what life was like for my grandmother. I got to thinking only 10 percent of her heart was working, she couldn't eat what she wanted, and she was always in pain. She fought hard to stay alive for us. She was supposed to have died years before when I was about 6. The doctors had us come and say our last goodbyes and everything, but somehow she pulled through. Her health was very bad. I liked to think she especially stayed around for me. She was the only person in my family that truly understood me and loved me unconditionally for who I was. She was my conscience and strength. At the end of the service I had to go and tell the pastor thank you and ask god for his forgiveness. From *that day on I made a vow that nothing would ever shake the faith I had in god ever again. That night I had an opportunity to reflect on things. I made up my mind to try to be less selfish (put a person who was worse off than me before me always) and look for a positive light in a bad situation. When I made it to work on Monday I felt like a changed person. My boss even noticed the difference. I was happier and more relaxed. I had become the person I was before I lost my grandmother. My boss wanted me around her most of the time, because of the attitude change and it was easier to talk to me now. She had the other two girls up front taking care of customers when she wanted me to hang with her in the back or go on company business. The girl Brenda who was the manager before my other co-worker Erica and I came to the store didn't like it. She and the main boss Darlene started bumping heads more. Mainly, because Erica became manager and Darlene liked hanging with me. When I changed weird things began to happen to me at work. The first time it happened I tried to unlock the door to the store. It wouldn't unlock and my key got jammed. I took out the key. I was about to put it back in, when the door unlocked on its own. I stood there for a minute before entering the door. I couldn't believe what just happened to me. When I went in the door I asked Brenda did she unlock the door and hurry back to her desk. She said no and when I went to the back no one was there. I told Erica what happened and she said I was crazy. I began to have these weird dreams as if I was one of the girls and I could see the murderers coming in the back door, I was seeing and going through everything they did. When I was about to see the faces of the murderers I would wake up. I don't know if this makes me crazy, but some of the most peaceful sleep I had was in that back office where those girls got murdered. When one of us was sick Darlene would tell us to lie down for a little while until we felt better. We didn't know we were lying in the same spot where the girl's bodies were laying when they were found. We didn't find that out until the DA and the defendants attorneys came back to the store to get measurement of the back office for the trial. Then Darlene decided to tell us that it was blood stains still on the floor under the carpet where they couldn't get it up. The thing about working at a loan company you run into a lot of different people and you hear a lot of their problems. I had customer come in at the last minute to pay on his loan. He got to telling me that he just came from his cousin's funeral. His cousin's mistress killed him. He had a wife; he chose to move in with the mistress. When he went to sleep one night, the mistress found out he was still sleeping with his wife and shot him in the head. All I could say, was sorry to hear that. They would just start telling their business hoping to get more money. I also had a woman con me out of $600. Luckily I was close to Darlene and she didn't fire me. She just had me pay the money back a little at a time. The woman also conned Brenda out of money too. We questioned her about it the next time she came in. She got nervous and starting coughing, because she and I got into an argument. I was* *sent to the back, because I was about to fight the woman. She couldn't stop coughing and Erica came to the back to get her some water. Darlene and I said get it out of the toilet at the same time. Erica didn't of course. I was still going to church so I handled the situation better than I would have if I hadn't been going. From that day on I refused to wait on her. The other girl's did. She stopped coming for awhile after we got into it and we let her know we caught on to her scheme. Everything was going fine in the office until Brenda started to do things behind our backs. She would mess with Erica until she would cry. One day Erica decided to go back to being a teller, because Brenda was picking on her. She wanted her old position back. She didn't mess with me, because she knew I would talk crazy to her back. I would feel sorry for Erica and stepped in and talked on her behalf. Darlene was watching all of this and was about to fire Brenda. Brenda knew she was going to be fired, because she got caught causing conflict between offices and she wasn't doing her job. The next morning she had come in and asked Darlene to talk in private. She told Darlene something very devastating and knew if Darlene fired her she could use it as a lawsuit. Darlene knew it too. She called me and Erica into the back after she sent Brenda home, because she was acting distraught and couldn't focus. She told us to be careful, because of what Brenda told her. I told them I already knew. Brenda told me as soon as I started working there. Erica got angry at me for not telling her, but Darlene understood why I didn't. I could have easily been sued too. Needless to say she didn't get fired. She went behind Darlene back and called the home office and told them the story too. The main office wanted Darlene to move to that office, because they said she was too close to us. Before Darlene left she made sure Brenda got moved to another store and Erica took back over as manager. She said she wouldn't feel right if she left me and Erica stuck with Brenda. Home office was keeping track of everything Brenda was doing. She didn't know, but we did. A couple of months later she got fired. She felt she beat them to the point they couldn't fire her. She got careless and made a lot of mistakes, so they had plenty of legitimate reasons to fire her. My aunt Terri insisted that we hire my uncle Donovan's girlfriend June. Since we didn't really feel like interviewing a lot of people we went ahead and hired her. June would always ask me why I was doing the extra work that I wasn't being paid for. I would go to different stores and do the job of the manager when I was only a cashier. I would fix the computers and paperwork and whatever else needed to be done. I would respond to her that I was getting all skills I could even if I was not being paid. I wasn't trying to impress anyone I just loved to learn and fix things most people can't. June was partially doing her job. Most of the time she was online, I do not know how she got into debt, but her drawer started coming up short. Erica was a nervous and scary person. She was afraid that if she told June she needed to put the money back in her drawer she would be mad and try to fight her. She was right, so I told her she* needed to put the money back in the drawer, because she was going to get us all fired. My aunt Terri would tell her I wouldn't put the money back they should have insurance on the money. She didn't realize this company didn't work like that. When I tried to explain it to her she didn't want to listen to me and because she didn't June didn't. I found out what I know personally. One day I hadn't cashed my check, because the banks and every place that cashed checks were closed. (The greedy owner extended the hours we worked from 9 a.m.- 6 p.m. To 9 a.m.-8 p.m . . He didn't care whether we had kids or if the neighborhoods were safe or not.) I called Erica and asked was it ok for me to borrow 5 dollars from the drawer to get gas so I could make it home. She told me to leave a note with my signature on it in my drawer. Luckily we had Darlene working at the main office in Texas she would give us a heads up when our new District Manager was coming. She had called Erica the next morning to tell her they were coming to our store for an audit. Erica didn't answer her phone right away, she got the call just as they were walking in the door. She called me and told me to hurry and get to work with the five dollars, because they were there. When I walked in the door to put my money back in the drawer the District Manager had just asked Erica why was there a note in my drawer for 5 dollars. We explained that I needed gas to get home, because I worked until closing and wasn't able to cash my check. She made a huge deal about the five dollars and told us we need to call and check with her before we do something like that. Then she asked me for the 5 dollars. I handed it to her and she continued her audit. A month later Darlene called us and told us to watch ourselves, because she heard the main people talking about something's she couldn't agree with. Not soon after that we got a phone call from Darlene saying she had quit so we needed to be very careful. Erica became even more nervous, because Darlene wasn't there to watch over us anymore and June was messing up. I wasn't so worried like Erica was, because I was going to church. That is when June's jealousy really kicked in. She started telling my boyfriend men were talking to me and she started calling in to work all the time. She was angry the men and customers wanted me to wait on them. I did my job quick when they needed me too and I didn't throw myself at the men. What made her really angry was the water guy Matt. While we were at work he would come on to Erica and me. We made it clear to him that we were taken. June was also, but she wanted him. People would tell us they saw her at RHJ High School on the weekends. That is where Matt practiced with his football team on the weekends. I never told my uncle what she was doing, because he was doing the same. One afternoon I was outside smoking a cigarette and June came running out of the store screaming. I asked her what was wrong she said it was a snake in the store by the computer towers. When I went in to check it out it was a baby water moccasin. I told Erica to stay and keep an eye on it while I called around for someone to come get it. She was the only one not afraid. Just as I was *calling animal control the lady that conned Brenda and me out of the money returned to the store for a loan. I didn't want to wait on her so I told June to. She had to reapply since it had been so long from her last loan her account closed. Her income had changed, so she got less money. She wasn't happy with it, so she started talking crazy to June. By this time the animal control man had made it. Erica and I were in the back with him. He grabbed the snake and as he did June came and got Erica about the customer. Just as Erica began talking to the lady the animal control man was walking to the door with the snake. June ran ahead of us, to open the door. The lady was so intent on getting more money out of Erica she never noticed the snake slithering toward her on the stick.*

Chapter Fourteen

It was 2002 and it seemed like the longer I went to church the weirder things began happening to me. I would be sitting at work alone and the toilet would start flushing on its own, things would go missing, and I began to see people in the spirit. I mentioned earlier about four girls murder. I went to school with one of them and my sisters went with the other three. They were shot in the head execution style. After they were shot the building was burned and so were three of them. Their spirits would mess with me so much to the point when I wasn't in the mood to deal with it. I would yell and tell them I wasn't in the mood to play with them. I was working one Saturday alone and I was smoking in the back. The chime went off on the door, so I put my cigarette out and went to the front. I took my lighter with me and sat it in front of my computer. It was my sister Karen bringing my nephew to see me, since I was always at work. When they left, I went to get my lighter and it was gone. I looked everywhere for it. I just gave up and said maybe my nephew took it when I let him in to use the bathroom. I closed the store down and went to get another one across the street. Monday when I made it to work Erica was fussing at me as I was walking through the door. She told me she had warned me about where I put my lighters. I asked her what she meant. She said as she was pulling her paperwork out and my lighter fell out of it. I told her the truth that I didn't put it there. I explained to her that I had left it in front of my computer and then it disappeared. I told her to call the other store and ask one of the girls if I called and told them I was shutting the store down for a couple of minutes to run and get something to eat. I didn't go get anything to eat I went to get a lighter I said to her. When we told June what had happened she started saying the same thing. The toilet flushed by itself. The funniest thing was when she said she had her purse and couldn't find it and then it magically appeared in the bathroom. We were laughing at her, because we saw her take her purse in the bathroom. When the anniversary of the murders came, I was looking out the window and I saw an older woman at the memorial site cleaning it. I decided to take her a broom, dust pan, and trash bag. When I started talking to her it turned out she was one of the girl's grandmother. I told her that I went to school with her granddaughter and she started telling me how much she missed her so much and at the time she was murdered she was the only grandchild she had. She said that they finally got another granddaughter and they sometimes call the little girl her other granddaughter name, because she looks just like her and act like her. She also started going into details about how she was frustrated with the media, because they keep saying her granddaughter was also burned beyond recognition. She said she wasn't that she fought when she was shot in the head the first time, so they shot her in the head again. She did not die. she was still crawling. They then shot her again. Where she was laying the ceiling fell on her after they set the building on fire, which preserved her body. When she finished talking I told her about all the weird things that were happening to me and she started laughing and said that sounds like those girls up to their old tricks. She gave me a hug and wished me well. I ended up getting in trouble by the District Manager, because one of the girls from the other store came while I was outside talking to the lady and told the District Manager on me. (Now you can see why I feel they hid my lighter.) While I was at church they told me that the closer I get to God the more I was going to see things in the spirit. I thought they were playing with me until I saw it for myself I started seeing the bad spirits people carried, instead of their faces. If they were ok I saw their face. June's features were that of a serpent. The cobra and then one day she stuck out her tongue and it too was shaped like a snake's tongue without the slit in it. I began to notice the difference in a lot of people and began to distance myself from the ones who didn't mean me any good. I slowly began to forgive the people who I felt I had done me wrong. The pastor had a sermon about forgiveness he said if we want god to forgive us then we need to forgive those who had hurt us. I forgave my father and bought him clothes after I told him how I felt about the abuse he did to my siblings and me. I took it a step further when my sister Karen told me about Tonya being abused by her boyfriend. I found her and talked to her. She told me how he beat her so bad that she lost the second baby she was carrying by him. He caused her to lose her child over a Butterfinger candy bar. She then told me she can't have anymore children, because of him. Her uterus is too damaged to carry a baby. I asked her would I ever let a man beat me she said no. Then I said to her why is she. I left before he came home. The next time I talked to her she said one day he came home while she was ironing her son's clothes and began to hit her, she took the hot iron and began hitting him with it. This time he went to the hospital. She eventually left him and is doing ok for herself. I even forgave Ethan's mom, and Holly. You see they made each time I went to court hell. Even though I forgave them I couldn't be around them, because they haven't changed. I had yet to forgive Ethan, I blamed him for a lot of things it was hard to.

Chapter Fifteen

As I was sitting at a fellow church member house waiting for her to finish doing my cousin's hair, her granddaughter was talking to me. Out of nowhere, in the conversation the little girl told me now you're free. I looked at her puzzled, her grandmother said, girl take it as a message, she is a prophetess in training. I did just that went on and didn't worry about the little girl saying that to me again. I started going to massage school a little after that. I went there full time. That meant I had to adjust my schedule at work so I could do them both. I met a lot of people while I was at school. When it came to the Academic part I past every test with an A or B. We had to do 150 hours of actual massages. I was one of the best in my class. When people would do their evaluation of me I got the highest score you get except twice. A pregnant woman wanted me to do a deep tissue massage and you can't do that. I explained to her that I could send her into early labor if I stimulated her body too much. The other was an Asian woman she always came in and never wanted to take her clothes off. She wanted a deep tissue massage and it was hard to do that without lotion and clothes on. She literally yelled at me to do it harder so I did. She yelled harder and I dug in with my fist as hard as I could then she said oy oy oy that hurt that hurt. I did it softer. Then she yelled even louder at me this time harder. I did it even harder. That went on like that for an hour. At the end of the session she gave me all ones. There were also five that made me feel so good about what I was doing. The first one was a body builder. I was praying that I didn't get her. I ended up getting her anyways. After I finished massaging her she came looking for me. She told me that she had been all over the world and had professional and amateur people massage her. She said that I was the best massage therapist she had in the whole twenty years. Then there was this older lady. Elderly people skin feels different, so I had to be more careful with her. It felt like her muscles was separate from her body. I was gentle with her though. When I came back in the room after they got dressed she tried to pay me. I told her thank you, but I can't take that. Her daughter got angry with me. She told me, I was offending her mom. I let her know since I didn't have a license I couldn't take money or I would never be able to get my license in this state. Sometimes the Health and Human Services will send people to see if we would take the money. Next was a lady that worked at the Wild Life Preserve. She told me that I found my true calling from god. Then it was this lady who always came to the school when they were giving massages for 10 dollars. She got up from the table and got dressed she told me that I was the best massage therapist she had since she had been getting them. I went to lunch. When I made it back she was yelling and waving to me when she seen me. She had been asking my teacher where I was and she specifically wanted me to massage her husband. She had told him that I was a great massage therapist and he didn't believe her. When he got up he was very relaxed. She told him you see what I mean, she is great isn't she. He told her I was. The last one was a customer of mine from my job girlfriend. He told me one day that she was having a hard time sleeping and the baby was giving her a hard time. He wanted to take her to dinner and a movie, but it was very hard for her to relax. I told him to bring her down to my school so I could give her a massage. When he brought her she was very tense. By the time I was done she had fallen to sleep on the table. He took her home to take a shower so they could go on their date she just wanted to sleep. He thanked me and told me that she hadn't been able to sleep that good in months. I like to think that I did great massages, because I put every ounce of energy that I had in them. While I was going to school my schedule was like this. I went to work in the morning, then got off, picked my daughter up from home, took her down to my mom's job and gave her to my mom and Derek, went to massage school for 6 hours, picked my daughter from my mom's, took her home, put her in the bed, then went to check on my boyfriend, went back home, and went to bed myself. I never stopped to think about problems June was causing Erica at work. Erica made a decision to take over being the manager at one of our other stores. She said she couldn't take working with June anymore. June wasn't listening to anything that Erica or I had to say she was risking our jobs with all the things she was doing. Erica had four children to think about so she left the store. When she left that meant we needed a manager at our store. I didn't know Erica suggested to our District Manager to promote me. When I found out about it I told them no. June wanted the position. I didn't want the responsibilities that Erica had. June made it impossible to be a good manager. Erica left so that meant until we found someone to replace her we had to do double shifts. June called in all the time so I ended having to work 6 days a week 16 hours a day. I didn't have time to see my family at all. One day Erica and the District Manager decided to trick me into coming to her office like there was something wrong with the computers there. I went to fix the computers, but nothing was wrong with them. When I got there, they told me it was important I take the position. They told me I had the skills and I was already doing the job of the manager I might as well take the job. I told the District manager I wanted to finish massage school and she told me I could it wouldn't interfere with my schooling. When I made it back to the office I told June I took the position and she got angry. The next step was to hire someone to take my job. Erica and I set up interviews. While we were interviewing June was talking crazy, because she was stuck up front waiting on customers. We interviewed an older woman. The interview lasted 20 minutes. We could tell eventually she would have a problem taking orders from a 23 year old woman. The next woman was the same age as me and we went to school together. We hit it off real good. The interview lasted maybe an hour or two. When she left June's comment was it was not fair we interviewed her longer than the older woman. We tried to explain to her the older woman was not going to take orders from me. Not only that she was too old to be working in a money place late at night, where people already have been murdered. She didn't have the experience working in loans. I think that June didn't want the younger girl there, because it meant competition in her eyes. Before we called Jasmine to come work for us I had to out of town to a manager meeting to the main office here in Texas. While I was in Dallas June was calling the other stores and telling the employees we weren't in Dallas at a meeting we were riding around having fun. The employees at the other stores told their managers what she was doing. They called me and told me to watch my back with her. The following Monday Jasmine started. I showed her what to do. I explained to her as long as she do her job and not cause any trouble she wouldn't have me in her face. She said I can work with that. She kept her end of the bargain up. She would bring me coffee in the morning and if I needed something done she was on it. She caught on pretty quick. When I was outside smoking she would come outside too. We would talk about the basketball team we were on together and everything else. She told me about her private life and then she asked me about June dating my uncle. She said June would be talking to other men on the phone and wanted her to match her with some of the men she was dating or had dated. I told her I try to stay out of that, because it is just going to lead to some huge drama. Then she met Matt. He was flirting with her while June was there. June got angry. The next morning Jasmine came in smiling. She told me she had sex with Matt the night before. I was shocked, because she had just met him. I told her not to get her heart involved with him, because was married and he tried to pin me in the corner and touch me, and that I think he was messing with June. I didn't say anything in front June about it, because I had this weird feeling. They both wanted him, he had these huge muscles and he was very cute. The next time he came in he told me about him and Jasmine. He said that her son was too bad for him and he couldn't be in a relationship with her. I told him that he shouldn't lead her on then. Then out of nowhere he said don't tell June, because she was going to be angry. I was wondering why she would be mad. He is just the water guy. For about a month I didn't worry *about them, because I was trying to get my money from all the overtime I had done, before we hired Jasmine. I was also trying to see why they didn't change my salary yet. When Matt came in for that month's water, he and Jasmine was flirting with each other in front of June. She was boiling mad. She asked me what was going on between them. I told her, you are a grown woman you know. Then she ask did they sleep together. I told her yes. All she said was she is h** and he would mess with anything. A couple of weeks later the radio station started having a contest where you can win this large amount of money. For the last two years June has been trying to win it, but didn't. Jasmine was very lucky she played the pick 3 of the lottery and hit at least once a week. One Friday it was Jasmine's turn to close on Friday. She called the radio station and won. Then she got her paycheck and also hit $600 dollars on the pick 3. She called me screaming she won. I told her she didn't, she said turn on the radio and I did. Sure enough they were saying her name. All I could do was tell her congratulation. I forgot to tell her to watch her back with June. The following Monday she told June she won the radio contest and June heard her name on the radio. She had this attitude all week long I didn't bother asking her what was wrong, because I knew. When we were at home, she would talk bad about Jasmine and I would take up for her. My aunt Terri didn't like it. When I left work that Wednesday everything was fine. Both cashiers money was there and the money that needed to be deposited for that evening was there. I made it in to work the next morning. The drawers was fine, all the money was there. The problem was the money order and western money was gone. That was about 3,000 dollars. I looked everywhere that I could think of in the store for the money. I was really trying to put off calling the District Manager. I knew they were going to find a way to blame me for the money being lost. Darlene had already given me the heads up about how they were. When I called them on Friday she immediately started blaming me and yelling at me. She came to our office and began to question everyone. Everyone said that when I left all the money was there. That left only Jasmine and June. Instead of her calling the police she just let us work the next 2 days. She had one of the other managers that I thought was one of my best friends call and get all our security information so they could change it. It was a 3 day weekend, because we weren't open on the 4th of July. When I made it in Tuesday morning the District Manager was there. She told me we were all fired. I told her that was wrong for them to do that to me. I never stole anything from them and I come to work every day, without missing a day for 3 years straight. I asked her when was I going to get my pay for being the manager, she told me that I didn't last past my probation period so I wouldn't get it. She didn't tell me there was a probation period before I took the position. When she said that I asked when was I going to get my overtime pay for all those days and hours I worked extra, she told me I wasn't. I called Jasmine and June and told them to go and get* *their belongings, because we got fired. As soon as I walked through the door to outside I heard the little girls' voice as if she was right there now you're free. I felt this huge weight lifted off my shoulders. I immediately went to Equal Employment office. I told them the whole story about them firing me even though both employees said when I left the money was there. I didn't know they could help me with getting my overtime pay and vacation pay so I didn't say anything about that. I just wanted to make sure they didn't give me a bad reference when I looked for another job and I could get my unemployment until I found another job. They lied and told the Equal Employment people they downsized, so they couldn't give me a bad reference or deny my unemployment. I then took my free time with my family and my daughter. I didn't have to go to school, because I graduated a couple months earlier. When I was looking for another job June came to me and asked did I want to look for jobs with her. I looked her in her eyes and told her I would never work with her again in this lifetime. She convinced my family Jasmine stole the money I knew different. Then one day her cousin got angry at her and told it that she was the one that stole the money and got us fired. I let my aunt Terri know exactly how I felt, because she was the one who told me to hire her. She ended getting arrested for something else and is not able to keep a steady job.*

Chapter Sixteen

Everything was going fine until I got hurt and almost died on January 20, 2004, a few days before my job interview with the county. My left knee got dislocated and almost severed my main artery in my leg. I was rushed to 2 different hospitals. I learned I have to wear a brace on my leg for the rest of my life. I was laid up for six months and couldn't do anything, but concentrate on my daughter school work. She was doing great, except when I signed paperwork for her to take gifted, talented classes, but she sabotage the test. I didn't know that at the time, because she starting daydreaming and her grades starting falling. I found out she needed glasses. I took her to get them. I healed and I got things in order with her teachers. The next school year she started off great then she fell back into her pattern. She wasn't being challenged enough. I punished her when she brought home an F in math. Next thing I know she got first place at her school science fair and first place at the state science fair, and by the last couple of months of school she was teaching the math class. I wanted her teacher to put in for her to go to a magnet school, but he said that she was not ready to go to that kind of school, because she was not motivated enough and they didn't put her in any pre-ap classes. The following day I went to the middle school they were going to send her to and talked to the lady that was going to be her counselor the next year. I requested that she be put in all pre-ap classes. We went into the next school year not knowing what to expect. The first year that she was there she made some awesome decisions on her own. She signed up for a program that changed our lives for the better called, Breakfree. When she took her state exams that are required for everyone to pass to the next grade, she got commended on all of them and on the math she scored higher than anyone in her grade. We got so many different offers from programs that would help her with college. Duke University even paid for her to take the ACT test in the seventh grade. She got nervous on the test and didn't do so well (it wasn't too bad to be a 7th grader). That didn't slow her down though. She was awarded the African American Heritage Award that year. One of the highest awards you can get in the School District. She was participating in so many *things and her grades were wonderful and she was first chair in band. She stayed on the honor roll and all the teachers and office staff knew who she was, heck they knew who I was, because she was so involved. She began going to UT at Austin for six weeks that summer with the Breakfree Program. I was more proud the next year my daughter was taking on so many different activities and keeping her grades up. The program that she chose to be in was helping us apply to different high schools that were more college level. One thing that I let my daughter know was that if things were too stressful for her that she can say when and we would cut some things out. The strong will that my daughter has she said no mom I can handle it. I left her alone and she showed me that she could. During this time I had to go to court with Ethan. We had to go to court, because he wasn't paying his child support. I made a decision then that I wouldn't hold a grudge on him anymore. He was in jail. Holly was still angry with me, so whoever she was on the phone with she was making jokes about me and Ethan being cousins and having sex. (We do not share the same gene pool anywhere.) I was about to cuss her out, but god works in mysterious ways. Just as she was about to sit down, she flipped over the side of the chair. The Sheriff and I both starting laughing, because he heard everything she was saying about me. He like the other Sheriff told me not to stoop to her level, because I was better than that, and he didn't want to arrest me. He said she deserved for me to kick her butt, but if I was to hit her first I would go to jail. When we went in front of the judge, she called Ethan and me first. She asked him why he wasn't paying child support at all to my daughter; he came up with a lot of excuses. The Judge told him he still needs to pay child support for my daughter. At the end of their conversation he told her I never come to him for anything. I just told the judge that my daughter needed money for all these extra things she is doing and sometimes I do need help. Even though I knew he had all this money I agreed to him paying $300 dollars to get out. I was tired of the arguing back and forth, so I just agreed. Then it was Ethan and Holly's turn. She was angry with him, she told the judge everything. She told the judge he got more money than he is saying and she wanted more than the $300 dollars he was offering to her. I just listened. 6 months later we were back in court and I told him how our daughter was doing in school. We actually had a civil conversation with each other instead of the arguing like we always did. He made a payment to the court for 300 dollars. I told Ethan what happened to Holly the last time we were in court and what she was saying about us right before she fell. I also told him how the sheriff was listening to her and said she deserved me to kick her butt. When we went in front of the judge I was like it doesn't matter what he pays, because I was tired of coming to court. I had been going for nine years. The judge hasn't done anything to him about not paying child support. I told her, I was just in a car accident. I wanted to sign the papers for him to get a probation officer and go. I couldn't leave, because I had to wait* *for the judge to hear Ethan's and Holly case so she could sign the paperwork for both cases at the same time. I listened how she was saying her bills cost more, because she included her child support in her income and he wasn't paying it. At the end when she and Ethan stopped arguing, she still didn't get the amount of money she wanted. Since she threatened to drop the kids off on him and leave them, he told her to bring them on. He had no problem taking care of his kids. While we were waiting in a room for them to bring our paperwork I told him she is crazy. He asked me why I said that. I told him the truth, there is no way in hell I would use child support as an income, because I know I am not going to get it. He looked at me like you know you are talking about me and I am right here. He didn't say it though. Instead he started flirting with me. I don't know how he knew, but he knew that I hadn't had sex in a long time. I asked him how he knew, he said because I know you. I didn't hear from him for awhile after that day. A few months after I went to court with Ethan my daughter's principal called me. I was shocked when the principal personally asked if my daughter could speak on the behalf of the school to the school board to keep it open. I thought it would be a one time thing, but every time there was a meeting the principal wanted my daughter there to speak. The last six weeks of school came. I was told my daughter was the Valedictorian. She gave a wonderful speech at the awards assembly. Later that day Ethan called me and told me that he was there. When I told my daughter she was very upset, because she felt he did not deserve to be there, she did not want him there, I told her, it was ok as long as he didn't approach her. She also received the African American Heritage Award that year too. We got a chance to see Maya Angelou in person with the help of Breakfree. She finished her summer program at UT with Breakfree, so she thought. She decided she wanted to be in the Battle of the Bands of 2008 at the beginning of summer. It is a huge competition from bands all over Texas. The day of the competition was also our family reunion. Ethan and his family showed up there. They thought they were going to see my daughter, but they didn't. He asked where were we and my cousin Emily told him where we were. They won second, but it should have been first. Most of the judges were from Houston, so you can guess who won. They were marching off the field my daughter spotted Ethan and his mom. She went into a panic mode and nearly ran into the street but she calmed down enough to stay in line. As soon as they made it back to the building she immediately ran where I was. She was literally having a panic attack. I asked her what was wrong she told me she saw Ethan and his family. I was furious He just showed up and didn't check to see if it was okay with me nor my daughter. That following Monday I called a child support lawyer. At first he and I were going back and forth arguing with each other, because neither of us understood what the other was meaning. Then I calmed down and began to really listen to him. He told me that if the judge didn't specifically put in the court order that he couldn't go to any of her programs then he can go as long as he didn't approach her. I called and I told him that she was quite upset about him just showing up. He thought it was me of course, but it wasn't. I was angry, because my daughter was so scared and couldn't breathe. I asked could we come to an agreement, so he does not just show up. I would call him to keep, him informed about everything she was doing. He told me that it wasn't the same. I understood that, but that is what she wanted. I asked her why was she so afraid of him. She brought up him fighting Holly in front of her, him on central Texas most wanted, and him getting shot. She said that it was from him selling drugs. For years I have been trying to explain why he ended up selling drugs to her, but she sticks to he should have gotten a job. I didn't know she remembered him fighting Holly, she didn't buy that it was a mistake that he was on the central Texas most wanted for assault, and she didn't care he got shot. He thinks my family and I sit around and talk about him to my daughter, but we don't. I talk to her to let her know one day she is going to have to talk to him. She told me she formed her opinion of him, because of him.*

Chapter Seventeen

My daughter got accepted in every high school she applied to one was a science academy, two were private schools, and one was a college level public school. She chose one of the private schools it is one of the most prestigious schools in the world. In the beginning at the new school was hard on her. She went from a kid that was the center of attention to one that was invisible. Things began to change for us around the same time school started. The man I had dated for ten years decided that he wanted to cheat. He listened to his mother and sisters and tried to date his ex girlfriend. I went to his house at 4 in the morning before, he went work. I asked him was he sure, because he is kind of mentally slow. He didn't know that I had this back up plan. He thought by time he got back from Houston he was going to change his mind if things didn't work out. He also thought that it was going to take awhile for me to get my belongings. His whole entire house was furnished with my things. He was cocky and said yes I'm sure. I said ok and then left. I put my daughter on her van to school and went back to his house. I called Ethan I explained to him that we broke up and I need him to come and get my stuff. He said give me 15 minutes and I'll be there. Sure enough 15 minutes later he drove up. As he drove up so did my sister Mary. When he walked up to me he, he asked, what did he do to you to make you mad. Ethan knows you have to do something to me to get me angry. I told him whatever he wanted he could have. He said can I have you. My response was we'll talk about that when we were alone. He and my sister moved all my things in the garage that I didn't give them, because he needed help to get my things. He told me he would be back later to get my stuff. I took that time to go get storage. When I made it back over there my ex boyfriend was home. I let him know that he didn't have to go outside at all when Ethan gets there, because I made sure that it was no reason for them to cross paths. He thought I was going to sit and hold a conversation with him as if he did nothing. He was still acting tuff, he said, he was sure this is what he wanted to do. While he was in mid sentence I saw Ethan's lights on his truck. I got so happy when I seen him I don't know why, that I got up and left my ex talking. Before I went out the door I told him not to come outside, because there was no reason for him to. He did anyway. Ethan, Garrett, and their friend was courteous and spoke to him even though they didn't want to. He heard Ethan tell me that he loved me. I did not hear him though. I was too busy catching up with Garrett, because I hadn't seen him in awhile. When I was finished talking to Garrett, Ethan, and me were under each other talking. They picked up a box that had all my idol merchandise in it. They began teasing me and asking do I still like Whitney. Garrett asked who stuff was in one of the tubs, I told him his niece. He got serious and told their friend he better not drop it or break anything in it, he was going to kick his butt. When Garrett finished talking, we all began talking about the past. My ex tried to break in the conversation and they were being nice, because it was his house and talked to him. Ethan barely said a word to him though until he said something stupid. He got to bragging about his temper tantrums, being violent, and destructive. Ethan gave him this look I have never seen before. He said, I hope you were not acting like that while my baby was around, while rubbing his chin.(of course I said it nicer) All my ex could do is have a stupid look on his face and started stuttering. I immediately told Ethan she was never around him while he was like that. (That is the truth, because my temper is just as bad as Ethan's if he hurt my daughter.) Only then did he relax. It is not like I hadn't warned my ex about Ethan. I had been telling him for years Ethan had a temper and he was very protective over his daughter. He thought I was lying, because Ethan was hardly in the picture. To this day my ex swears he didn't' hear Ethan say that and he was a foot away from him. Ethan decided only to make one trip that night. He said that he would come back the next night to remove the rest of my stuff. Instead it was 2 nights later he got caught up in doing a moving job. Ethan told me a couple of days before to give the furniture to goodwill. The day goodwill came. When my ex made it home he was furious, the whole house was empty. He realized that he lost me. He went into one of his tantrums and the whole neighborhood was watching him. So the neighbor had stopped me and begged me not to go in the house by myself when she seen me drive up. I told her it is fine he's at work. She said she was afraid that he might try to kill me, so when I come back later to get the rest of my stuff don't come alone. I explained that I was going to have some big men with me I'll be alright. We made it back to his house. Karen and Mary were with me. They were watching Ethan, how he was watching me and acting. The next door neighbor came out and I started talking to her. I told her see they some big dudes and we started laughing. I told her who Ethan was. Ethan was watching me even then. I called him over and introduced him to her and he gave her his business card. He then went and started talking to my sisters. When he left us the neighbor said he loves you very much, you can tell. When we left to take my last load to storage my ex was in the driveway looking sad. I followed Ethan to the storage and when they finished unloading my stuff he began to tell me how much he loves his daughter and me. That I didn't owe him anything he just wants to see his daughter. He thought that I was lying when I told him I had to see how she felt, before I agreed to it. He reluctantly agreed and we left. I told my daughter what he said. She told me just, because he helped you does not mean I have to deal with him, that's you. I told him what she said and he wanted to know what he did to make her not want to deal with him. I told him what she told me that she was afraid of him, because she remembers seeing his picture in the newspaper saying "WANTED" and she remembered him hitting Holly. She also said that he made her get a blood test and that he haven't been there. I told him every word she said and he said I need to let the past go. That is what your daughter said, he still didn't believe me.

Chapter Eighteen

I had even less to worry about with my ex out of the picture. My daughter was about to lose one of her mentors in the Breakfree program. Jim decided to quit to become a teacher. She and he were close. That was going to be his last year. She struggled with her grades and she didn't have but a couple of friends. Her school paid for her a tutor. We also went to the Breakfree program's office for tutoring. She made it through to the next grade barely. She told me that the 2010-2011 school year will be better. We got to record a video for a program, that supports higher education for the state of Texas. they interviewed the governor and a lot of very important people too. I emailed Ethan the website. My daughter was angry, because they cut a lot of her talking out. That summer she went to UT for a few weeks instead of six like normal. Our family reunion came when my daughter was available so we went. Everything was going great. While I was sitting outside Ethan and his family drove up. My daughter was in the building listening to music and playing with some of her cousins. The kids went inside and told her that he was outside. I text her when he was outside, so they couldn't make it seem worse than it was. I received a text from her, why with a lot of exclamation marks. I guess I text too slow, because she called me while I was texting her back. I couldn't hear anything that she was saying. She got frustrated and started yelling through the phone for me to unlock the door. I told her it was already unlocked. Next thing I know she bolted right past me and jumped in the car. Ethan and his mom saw this and he got angry and she started crying. He started yelling saying, his daughter don't have to be hiding in a hot car. If it would take for him to leave for her to come out the car, he would leave. His mom was crying saying something about how it hurts, how her granddaughter is hiding in the hot car from them. I really didn't understand what she was saying, because she was crying. Then she started blaming someone about how my daughter responded, I thought she was talking about me. So I said I had nothing to do with her running to the car. She and Ethan said at the same time in a reassuring way we not talking about you. Jaime, Derek, my uncle Larry, and my aunt Suzanne was right there. Jaime said I know you are not talking about me. Ethan and his mom started talking again and I can't remember what they said. Derek and I told Jaime to be quiet. She did, for a little while. Next thing I know Ethan starting talking even louder and said that no one has the say so with what goes on with our baby, but me and him. He then started saying, because it was me and him sneaking in those hallways. Up until he got to that part I let him blow off his steam. I gave him this look and put my finger up, as I did this I told lets go over here and talk by ourselves, because he is getting to personal with my private life. When we made it to a private area, he broke down and started crying. He told me that I don't know how it feels not to be able to talk to or see your child. I told him actually I do. I have to say to him I apologize for saying I do, because I don't. He said he doesn't understand what his mom has done to my daughter. I told him do you remember when you hired that lawyer. He said yes. I told when you went to the bathroom your mom and Holly was calling me out of my name while she was sitting there. That she got so angry that she tried to throw her shoes at the both of them. I told him that is why my family went to their house. He didn't say anything about what I had just said. I explained to him that when I tried to hang with his sister, so he could develop some kind of relationship with her he wasn't ready. He wanted to hang with his friends and sell drugs. Now that she is older he is ready and she is not. They have me stuck in the middle with them not being on the same page. That he needed to give her, her space. When she is ready she would come around. I also took this opportunity to tell him again that all the things I would tell him in the past it was not me speaking it was her. He told me if she wanted him to leave he would, because he wanted her to be comfortable. I told him to let me go talk to her and see what she wants. (Now he knows why I would say let me talk to her first, before I agree for him to see her or talk to her.) As we were walking back to the car he told me she wasn't in there anymore. She ran around the corner. I asked him when she got out. That was the first time that I have seen that kid move that fast. I walked around the corner and found her. I told her he said if she wanted him to leave, he would. She told me as long as they didn't talk to her she was fine. When I went back to Ethan I told him word for word what she said. He said he could live with that. His baby said he can stay so what anybody else says doesn't matter to him. I told him if there is any trouble my daughter and I were leaving and we wouldn't be making it to anymore family functions. He said he wasn't going to do anything. Derek, Ethan, Garrett, and I were talking about the past having a good time. My daughter came and got me, because she wanted her book out of the car. When she got it Carrie approached her. She just looked at Carrie like she was crazy. When Carrie stopped talking to her I apologized to her about my daughter being rude. She told me it was okay, because all of Ethan's kids act just like him. Show exactly how they feel. Then she told my daughter she was going to give me her number, so she could call her whenever she wanted. She never gave it to me; I guess she figured my daughter would never call her. Jaime made sure that she made them as uncomfortable as she could. I prayed that they would over look her and they did, because I didn't wanted the family reunion ruined. Everyone was having a great time. I had Spot with me. That's the family dog. Ethan's mom asked me was he my dog. I told her no, but Derek said yes. Spot thinks that I am his mom, so I treat him like my baby. Ethan was impressed with the colors on his head, but he thought since he was small he would not do anything. He started making noises at him, to intimidate him. Derek said get him and Spot snapped at his hand. Ethan jumped back quick. Then his nephew came up to me and started talking to me. He asked did I used to babysit him. I told him yes. I enjoyed my conversation with him. Then I got to see Carrie's stepson who I had been asking about every time I saw his dad. I talked to Carrie's ex husband and told him that Carrie approached her, when she asked them not to. He said that they should just give her time and she would come around. I left that night a little confused. I was starting to feel like nothing bad has ever happened between Ethan and me. We even were entertaining the idea of us messing around again. Nothing ever came of that though. Ethan asked me again why his daughter doesn't want to deal with him. My ex boyfriend told me, he and my daughter sat at the front of the park waiting on Ethan, when she was 4. He never showed. When I asked my daughter she admitted to me that was true. She said Ethan was suppose had bought her some sidewalk chalk shaped like ice cream, and gave it to her that day. She say that he lies and don't keep his promises. She also mentioned that she want to know why he made her take a blood test and no one else. That was all that I could get out of her. I told Ethan what she said. He said that he had to explain it to her, why he did the things he did or didn't do. I suggested he write her a letter. Needless to say he did not. When her birthday came he called her, but her didn't get her anything. She said I or she shouldn't have to ask him for anything he should just do it. Since she had the free time during the summer she volunteered at the hospital she was born at, because at her school she has to do 12 hours of community service. She decided to get it over with during the summer, so she can do more activities during the school year.

Chapter Nineteen

It is now 2010-2011 school year. My daughter is a sophomore. The year started out fine. I had known since last school year she was going to be going to Italy. I needed to come up with $4,000 dollars. I told Ethan how much I needed, but he didn't try to help, I guess since I didn't or my daughter didn't ask him to help. I got loans and used some of the money that I had been saving up for my daughter to get her there. Even though he didn't help us I told him to get a passport, so if we needed we could just hop on a plane to get to her. He said he would, I think he was just saying ok to me. When I asked him later did he get one, he said no. I just went ahead and told him don't worry about it, if he had issues with the law. This year is her adventurous year, for winter sports she became manager of the soccer team since she isn't very interested in actually participating in sports. She offered to manage the girl's basketballs team but the coach already had two managers. One of her friends suggested soccer, so she offered to manage the boy's soccer team and she did really well and she was very dedicated. However, the school couldn't afford to take her to SPC Tournaments with them, so she had to stay but they had a great tournament anyway. Things settled down after the SPC Winter Sports for awhile, until March when she went off to Italy. She bragged that I would be the one crying, but when everyone was saying goodbye she started tearing up. I told her in a joking way you better suck it, because here come your friends. She fixed her face and went off to Italy for 10 days. My aunt Terri gave her an extra $500 dollars for spending money. In all she had about a $1,000 dollars to blow on whatever she wanted. Before she left she made sure she set up me a Skype account, so I could see her. I also bought her an international phone, so I could call her whenever I wanted. I called Ethan the night before she left. He asked could he go to the airport with us, but I told him no. Our daughter is still angry with him and refuse to see or talk to him. I ask him did he want me to let him know when she got back, he said yes. He also wanted to go with me to pick her up. Again I had to say no. When her plane landed I called Ethan, but he didn't answer the phone. When she got back she told me *how she went to the fashion capitol of the world and when she went to Verona the city famously known for Romeo and Juliet and went to see Juliet's house. She took a picture with the statue, but when I saw the picture I asked what she was doing. She explained that she didn't want to offend the Italians and she had to touch Juliet's breast for good luck in relationships. She also went to a carnival and bought a mask and celebrated with her friends. She went to a lot of Cathedrals which is good, because I feel it's important for her to learn about religions. In one of the Cathedrals, she saw the body of Pope John Paul 2; she said it was the first step for him to become a saint. She got to see the statue David by Michael Angelou. She brought back a lot of gifts for everyone. Recently she went to New Mexico for a festival for 4 days she just got back and she told me she had a lot of fun, because she made new friends and they invited her to their show and offered to help her play the electric guitar, because she's a rocker. While she was in New Mexico, I tried to meet with Ethan. I wanted to apologize to him about of a lot of the choices that I made for him instead of with him. He called me the day he was suppose to meet me. He said he had to do a moving job and he didn't know how long it was going to take. I let him know I would be home up until a certain time. I tried calling him and texting him for a couple of days to let him know our daughter made it home from New Mexico and to tell one of his sons Happy Birthday. I don't know if I would ever get the chance to apologize for making choices for him, instead of with him. I do know I did make the right choice, but it should have been with him. He did offer for her to use any of his six vehicles to learn how to drive in and to pay for her sweet 16 party. He is just waiting to see if she would come to him and ask him herself. I highly doubt she would, but only time can tell. I have the faith in my daughter that eventually she would gain the insight that I have and see that she is destined for great things. Not only is she wise beyond her years, she is very blessed, she would make the right choices in the end.*

www.ingramcontent.com/pod-product-compliance
Lightning Source LLC
Chambersburg PA
CBHW021242280526
45784CB00005B/2209